Geriatric Psychiatry

Editors

LOUIS J. MARINO, Jr
GEORGE S. ZUBENKO

PSYCHIATRIC CLINICS OF NORTH AMERICA

www.psych.theclinics.com

Consulting Editor
HARSH K. TRIVEDI

December 2022 • Volume 45 • Number 4

ELSEVIER

1600 John F. Kennedy Boulevard ● Suite 1800 ● Philadelphia, Pennsylvania, 19103-2899

http://www.theclinics.com

PSYCHIATRIC CLINICS OF NORTH AMERICA Volume 45, Number 4
December 2022 ISSN 0193-953X, ISBN-13: 978-0-323-93963-8

Editor: Megan Ashdown
Developmental Editor: Diana Grace Ang

Psychiatric Clinics of North America (ISSN 0193-953X) is published quarterly by Elsevier Inc., 360 Park Avenue South, New York, NY 10010-1710. Months of issue are March, June, September, and December. Business and Editorial Offices: 1600 John F. Kennedy Blvd., Suite 1800, Philadelphia, PA 19103-2899. Periodicals postage paid at New York, NY and additional mailing offices. Subscription prices are $345.00 per year (US individuals), $985.00 per year (US institutions), $100.00 per year (US students/residents), $414.00 per year (Canadian individuals), $509.00 per year (international individuals), $1005.00 per year (Canadian & international institutions), and $220.00 per year (international students/residents), $100.00 per year (Canadian & students/residents). Foreign air speed delivery is included in all Clinics' subscription prices. All prices are subject to change without notice. **POSTMASTER:** Send address changes to Psychiatric Clinics of North America, Elsevier Health Sciences Division, Subscription Customer Service, 3251 Riverport Lane, Maryland Heights, MO 63043. **Customer Service: 1-800-654-2452 (US). From outside the United States, call 1-314-447-8871. Fax: 1-314-447-8029. E-mail: journalscustomerservice-usa@elsevier.com (for print support) and journalsonlinesupport-usa@elsevier.com (for online support).**

Reprints. For copies of 100 or more, of articles in this publication, please contact the Commercial Reprints Department, Elsevier Inc., 360 Park Avenue South, New York, New York 10010-1710. Tel.: 212-633-3874, Fax: 212-633-3820, E-mail: reprints@elsevier.com.

Psychiatric Clinics of North America is covered in MEDLINE/PubMed (Index Medicus), Current Contents/Social and Behavioral Sciences, Social Science Citation Index, Embase/Excerpta Medica, and PsycINFO.

Contributors

CONSULTING EDITOR

HARSH K. TRIVEDI, MD, MBA
President and Chief Executive Officer, Sheppard Pratt, Clinical Professor of Psychiatry, University of Maryland School of Medicine, Baltimore, Maryland, USA

EDITORS

LOUIS J. MARINO Jr, MD
Medical Director, Geriatric Services, Sheppard Pratt, Baltimore, Maryland , USA; Associate Professor, Clinical, The Warren Alpert Medical School, Brown University, Providence, Rhode Island, USA

GEORGE S. ZUBENKO, MD, PhD
Distinguished Life Fellow, American Psychiatric Association, Fellow, American Association for the Advancement of Science, Washington, DC, USA; Fellow Emeritus, American College of Neuropsychopharmacology, Brentwood, Tennessee, USA

AUTHORS

SILPA BALACHANDRAN, MD
Assistant Professor of Psychiatry, Northeast Ohio Medical University, Adult and Geriatric Psychiatry, Cleveland Clinic-Akron General, Akron, Ohio, USA

KRIPA BALARAM, MD
Resident Physician, Department of Psychiatry, MetroHealth Medical Center, Case Western Reserve University School of Medicine, Cleveland, Ohio, USA

THOMAS A. BAYER, MD
Advanced Research Fellow, Long-term Services and Supports Center of Innovation, Providence VA Medical Center, Clinical Instructor, Division of Geriatrics and Palliative Medicine, The Warren Alpert Medical School, Brown University, Providence, Rhode Island, USA

DAVID M. CARLSON, MD
Psychiatry/Mental Health Service, VA Greater Los Angeles Healthcare System, Department of Psychiatry and Biobehavioral Sciences, David Geffen School of Medicine at UCLA, Los Angeles, California, USA

ZACHARY L. COHEN, MD
Yale School of Medicine, New Haven, Connecticut, USA

MICHELLE L. CONROY, MD
Assistant Professor of Psychiatry, Yale School of Medicine, New Haven, Connecticut, USA; VA Connecticut Healthcare System, West Haven, Connecticut, USA

COLEMAN K. COSGROVE, DO, PhD
Department of Psychiatry, University at Buffalo, Buffalo, New York, USA

LUCAS CRAWFORD-HOLLAND, BA
Keenan Research Centre for Biomedical Science, St. Michael's Hospital, Toronto, Ontario, Canada

CHRISTINA S. DINTICA, PhD
Department of Psychiatry, Neurology, and Epidemiology, University of California, San Francisco, San Francisco, California, USA

EBONY DIX, MD
Assistant Professor, Department of Psychiatry, Yale School of Medicine, New Haven, Connecticut, USA

PAUL M. EIGENBERGER, MD
Yale School of Medicine, New Haven, Connecticut, USA

ALISANDREA ELSON, MD
Department of Psychiatry, Creighton University School of Medicine, Omaha, Nebraska, USA

GARY EPSTEIN-LUBOW, MD
Associate Professor, Department of Psychiatry and Human Behavior, The Warren Alpert Medical School, Brown University, Associate Professor, Department of Health Services, Policy and Practice, Brown University School of Public Health, Staff Psychiatrist, Butler Hospital, Providence, Rhode Island, USA

CORINNE E. FISCHER, MD
Keenan Research Centre for Biomedical Science, St. Michael's Hospital, Department of Psychiatry, University of Toronto, Toronto, Ontario, Canada

NAREK HAKOBYAN, BSc
Keenan Research Centre for Biomedical Science, St. Michael's Hospital, Toronto, Ontario, Canada

DYLAN HERSHKOWITZ, MD
Clinical Instructor, Department of Psychiatry and Human Behavior, The Warren Alpert Medical School, Brown University, Providence, Rhode Island, USA

KELSEY A. HOLIDAY, PhD
Psychiatry/Mental Health Service, VA Greater Los Angeles Healthcare System, Los Angeles, California, USA

PALLAVI JOSHI, DO, MA
Banner Alzheimer's Institute, Department of Psychiatry, University of Arizona College of Medicine-Phoenix, Phoenix, Arizona, USA

CAITLIN LAWRENCE, MD
Assistant Professor, Department of Psychiatry and Human Behavior, The Warren Warren Alpert Medical School, Brown University, The Miriam Hospital, Providence, Rhode Island, USA

REBECCA J. MELROSE, PhD
Psychiatry/Mental Health Service, VA Greater Los Angeles Healthcare System, Department of Psychiatry and Biobehavioral Sciences, David Geffen School of Medicine at UCLA, Los Angeles, California, USA

DAVID G. MUNOZ, MD, MSc
Keenan Research Centre for Biomedical Science, St. Michael's Hospital, Department of
Laboratory Medicine and Pathobiology, University of Toronto, Toronto, Canada

ANDREW NAMASIVAYAM, MD
Department of Psychiatry, University of Toronto, Toronto, Ontario, Canada

NICOLÁS PÉREZ PALMER, MD
Department of Psychiatry, Yale School of Medicine, New Haven, Connecticut, USA

BRUCE G. POLLOCK, MD, PhD
Campbell Family Mental Health Research Institute, Division of Geriatric Psychiatry, Centre
for Addiction and Mental Health, Toronto Dementia Research Alliance, University of
Toronto, Toronto, Ontario, Canada

KAMOLIKA ROY, MD
Geriatric Psychiatry Fellow, Department of Psychiatry, Yale School of Medicine,
New Haven, Connecticut, USA

JAMES L. RUDOLPH, MD, SM
Director, Long-term Services and Supports Center of Innovation, Providence VA Medical
Center, Professor, Division of Geriatrics and Palliative Medicine, The Warren Alpert
Medical School, Brown University, Professor, Department of Health Services, Policy and
Practice, Brown University School of Public Health, Providence, Rhode Island,
USA

TOM A. SCHWEIZER, PhD
Keenan Research Centre for Biomedical Science, St. Michael's Hospital, Department of
Neurosurgery, University of Toronto, Toronto, Ontario, Canada

KATHERINE M. SHARKEY, MD, PhD, FAASM, FACP
Departments of Medicine, and Psychiatry and Human Behavior, The Warren Alpert
Medical School, Brown University, Providence, Rhode Island, USA

DEENA J. TAMPI, MSN, MBA-HCA, RN, DFAAGP
Co-Founder and Managing Principal, Behavioral Health Advisory Group, Princeton, New
Jersey, USA

RAJESH R. TAMPI, MD, MS, DFAPA, DFAAGP
Professor and Chairman, Bhatia Family Endowed Chair, Department of Psychiatry,
Creighton University School of Medicine, Omaha, Nebraska, USA

BARBARA TREJO ORTEGA, MD
Department of Psychiatry, Yale School of Medicine, New Haven, Connecticut, USA

LAURA I. VAN DYCK, MD
Mount Sinai School of Medicine, New York, New York, USA

RYAN VAN PATTEN, PhD
Clinical Neuropsychologist, Providence VA Medical Center, Assistant Professor,
Department of Psychiatry and Human Behavior, The Warren Alpert Medical School,
Brown University, Providence, Rhode Island, USA

ANGELA WANG, MD
Department of Psychiatry and Human Behavior, The Warren Alpert Medical School,
Brown University, Providence, Rhode Island, USA

KIRSTEN M. WILKINS, MD
Yale School of Medicine, New Haven, Connecticut, USA; VA Connecticut Healthcare System, West Haven, Connecticut, USA

KRISTINE YAFFE, MD
Department of Psychiatry, Neurology, and Epidemiology, University of California, San Francisco, San Francisco VA Health Care System, San Francisco, California, USA

BRANDON C. YARNS, MD, MS
Psychiatry/Mental Health Service, VA Greater Los Angeles Healthcare System, Department of Psychiatry and Biobehavioral Sciences, David Geffen School of Medicine at UCLA, University of California, Los Angeles, Los Angeles, California, USA

Contents

This review discusses the evolving evidence base and clinical considerations for examining the direct and indirect effects of the coronavirus disease (COVID-19) pandemic on the mental health of elderly individuals. It briefly addresses the cognitive and psychiatric outcomes in older adults who have survived COVID-19 infections and the complexity of appraising them during different stages of the pandemic. Indirect effects of the COVID-19 pandemic on the mental health of the geriatric population are also explored, including those influenced by quarantine, media campaigns, discrimination, and difficulties in accessing supportive services like long-term care and medical care.

Severe acute respiratory syndrome coronavirus 2, the novel coronavirus responsible for the coronavirus disease (COVID-19), affects the brain. Neurologic and neuropsychiatric symptoms may manifest in the acute and post-acute phases of illness. The vulnerability of the brain with aging further increases the burden of disease in the elderly, who are at the highest risk of complications and death from COVID-19. The mechanisms underlying the effects of COVID-19 on the brain are not fully known. Emerging evidence vis-à-vis pathogenesis and etiologies of COVID-19 brain effects is promising and may pave the way for future research and development of interventions.

Cognitive impairment and dementia affect dozens of millions of people worldwide and cause significant distress to patients and caregivers and a financial burden to families and health care systems. Careful history-taking, cognitive and physical examination, and supplemental neuroimaging and fluid-based biomarkers can accurately diagnose neurocognitive disorders. Management includes non-pharmacological and pharmacological treatments tailored to the etiology and to the individual.

> Alzheimer's disease (AD) is the most common neurodegenerative disease leading to dementia worldwide. While neuritic plaques consisting of aggregated amyloid-beta proteins and neurofibrillary tangles of accumulated tau proteins represent the pathophysiologic hallmarks of AD, numerous processes likely interact with risk and protective factors and one's culture to produce the cognitive loss, neuropsychiatric symptoms, and functional impairments that characterize AD dementia. Recent biomarker and neuroimaging research has revealed how the pathophysiology of AD may lead to symptoms, and as the pathophysiology of AD gains clarity, more potential treatments are emerging that aim to modify the disease and relieve its burden.

> In this article, the authors discuss primarily what is known about the epidemiology of all-cause dementia. Dementia is caused by a complex interplay of genetics, comorbidities, and lifestyle factors, and drug development has been challenging. However, evidence from large, prospective, observational studies has identified a variety of factors that may prevent or delay the onset of dementia. Several of these factors are modifiable and lend themselves to well to treatments currently available. The authors discuss the state of current evidence on dementia risk factors, the most promising avenues, and future directions for dementia prevention and management.

> This review covers the latest advances in our understanding of psychosis in the elderly population with respect to diagnosis, epidemiology, and treatment. Major topics of discussion include late life psychiatric disorders such as schizophrenia, schizoaffective disorder, and delusional disorder as well as dementia-related psychosis. Clinical differences between early-onset and late-onset disorders are reviewed in terms of prevalence, symptomatology, and approach to treatment. Newly revised research and clinical criteria for dementia-related psychosis are referenced. The evidence base for emerging therapies including citalopram and pimavanserin in relation to conventional therapies such as atypical antipsychotics are discussed.

> The population of elderly in the United States with substance use disorders (SUDs) is growing appreciably. SUDs among the elderly are often associated with poor outcomes and are frequently underdiagnosed. The current diagnostic criteria are less sensitive in identifying SUDs

among the elderly. Routine screening with validated screening tools may improve the diagnosis of SUDs among the elderly. There is a dearth of data from controlled studies on SUDs among the elderly and the use of pharmacologic agents for treatment, although data indicate that older adults with SUDs respond well to treatments that are specifically designed for this age group.

Sleep disruption is common in older adults and is associated with many poor health outcomes. It is vital for providers to understand insomnia and other sleep disorders in this population. This article outlines age-related changes in sleep, and medical, psychiatric, environmental, and psychosocial factors that may impact sleep. It addresses the evaluation of sleep symptoms and diagnosis of sleep disorders. It aims to examine the evidence for non-pharmacological and pharmacologic treatment options for insomnia while weighing factors particularly germane to the aging adult.

A growing percentage of the population is aging, with a large subset of this group meeting criteria for one or more neuropsychiatric disorders. Generally, physiological changes due to aging affect most of the pharmacokinetic processes in the body, with age-related physiologic changes in cardiovascular, gastric, hepatic, and renal function leading to changes in the pharmacokinetics of medications that can affect the absorption, distribution, accumulation, and clearance and elimination of various medications. This article aims to discuss the common pharmacodynamic and pharmacokinetic changes associated with physiologic aging and their impacts on the use of psychotropic medications in the elderly.

Aging increases susceptibility to medical and psychiatric comorbidity via interrelated biological, psychological, and social mechanisms. Mental status changes or other psychiatric symptoms occurring in older adults with medical disorders most often result from delirium, depression, or the onset of Alzheimer's disease and related dementias (ADRD). Clinicians can use evidence-based tools to evaluate such symptoms including the 4A's Test for delirium, the Saint Louis University Mental Status Exam, and the Geriatric Depression Scale. Innovative models such as collaborative care can improve the outcome of care of older adults with medical disorders requiring treatment for depression or ADRD.

The older adult population in the United States is poised to reach 83.7 million by 2050, and up to 20% will suffer from cognitive and mental illnesses. We do not have the workforce available to meet this need; therefore, general psychiatrists will care for many older psychiatric patients. Enhancing learning opportunities during general medical education and residency could improve the knowledge of general psychiatrists and encourage recruitment into geriatric psychiatry. This article outlines geriatric psychiatry education in medical school, residency, and geriatric psychiatry fellowship with suggestions for recruitment into the field, along with recommendations for enhanced learning for general psychiatrists.

PSYCHIATRIC CLINICS OF NORTH AMERICA

THE CLINICS ARE AVAILABLE ONLINE!
Access your subscription at:
www.theclinics.com

Preface

Geriatric Psychiatry

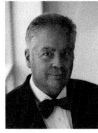 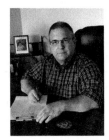

Louis J. Marino, Jr, MD   George S. Zubenko, MD, PhD
Editors

This issue of *Psychiatric Clinics of North America* on Geriatric Psychiatry includes 11 articles contributed by recognized experts who provide updates of their areas of clinical focus. Their contributions are greatly appreciated and presented in an order that enhances their readability and integration.

The article by Wang and Lawrence describes the "Impact and of SARS-CoV-2 Infections and Pandemic on Brain Function in the Elderly." This contribution provides a broad-based description of the pandemic with emphasis on the disproportionately high mortality among the elderly segment of the population, neuropsychiatric effects, and persistent longer-term complications (long-COVID). Multiple international organizations, including the WHO, CDC, and NIH, have recommended vaccination for eligible older adults to prevent and reduce the risk of severe illness.

The article, "Brain Effects," by Dix and Roy focuses on mechanisms by which SARS-CoV-2 infection affects the brain, including inflammation, neuroinvasion, microvasculature injury, and hypoxia. These insults may contribute to the neurologic and psychiatric symptoms during the acute and postacute phases of COVID-19, to which older adults are the most vulnerable. Early findings from the UK Biobank COVID-19 longitudinal case-control imaging study suggest greater reduction in global brain size, the possibility of the left cerebral hemisphere being more strongly associated with SARS-CoV-2 infection, and longitudinal limbic olfactory brain changes involving functionally connected regions of anterior cingulate cortex, orbitofrontal cortex, amygdala, hippocampus, and parahippocampal gyrus. These and related findings may foster the development of effective, targeted treatments for COVID-19 and other brain disorders.

In the article by Perez-Palmer and colleagues, "Cognitive Impairment in Older Adults: Epidemiology, Diagnosis, and Treatment" is addressed. Cognitive impairment and dementia affect dozens of millions of people worldwide, causes significant distress to patients and caregivers, and creates financial burden to families and health

Psychiatr Clin N Am 45 (2022) xiii–xvi
https://doi.org/10.1016/j.psc.2022.08.001
0193-953X/22/© 2022 Published by Elsevier Inc.

care systems. Careful history-taking, cognitive and physical examination, and supplemental neuroimaging and fluid-based biomarkers can accurately diagnose neurocognitive disorders. Management includes nonpharmacologic and pharmacologic treatments tailored to the cause and to the individual.

Next, Yarns and colleagues describe the "Pathophysiology of Alzheimer Disease." Alzheimer disease (AD) is the most common neurodegenerative process leading to dementia worldwide. While neuritic plaques consisting of aggregated amyloid-beta proteins and neurofibrillary tangles of accumulated tau proteins represent the pathophysiologic hallmarks of AD, numerous processes likely interact with risk and protective factors and one's culture to produce the cognitive loss, neuropsychiatric symptoms, and functional impairments that characterize AD dementia. Recent biomarker and neuroimaging research has revealed how the pathophysiology of AD may lead to symptoms, and as the pathophysiology of AD gains clarity, more potential treatments are emerging that aim to modify the disease and relieve its burden.

In Dinica and Yaffe's article, they address the "Epidemiology and Risk Factors for Dementia." The authors discuss the epidemiology of "all-cause" dementia. Dementia is caused by a complex interplay of aging, genetics, comorbidities, and lifestyle factors, and drug development has been challenging. However, evidence from large, prospective, observational studies has identified a variety of factors that may prevent or delay the onset of dementia. Several of these factors are modifiable and lend themselves to treatments currently available. The authors discuss the state of current evidence on dementia risk factors, the most promising avenues, and future directions for dementia prevention and management.

In the article by Fischer and colleagues, they discuss "Psychotic Disorders in the Elderly: Diagnosis, Epidemiology, and Treatment." This review covers recent advances in our understanding of psychosis in the elderly population with respect to diagnosis, epidemiology, and treatment. Major topics of discussion include late life psychiatric disorders, such as schizophrenia, schizoaffective disorder, and delusional disorder as well as dementia-related psychosis. Clinical differences between early-onset and late-onset disorders are reviewed in terms of prevalence, symptoms, and approach to treatment. Newly revised research and clinical criteria for dementia-related psychosis are referenced. The evidence for emerging therapies, including citalopram and pimavanserin, in relation to conventional therapies, such as atypical antipsychotics, is discussed.

Tampi and colleagues' article discusses "Substance Abuse Disorders in the Elderly." The population of elderly in the United States with substance use disorders (SUDs) is growing appreciably. SUDs among the elderly are often associated with poor outcomes and are frequently underdiagnosed. The current diagnostic criteria are less sensitive in identifying SUDs among the elderly. Routine screening with validated screening tools may improve diagnosis of SUDs among the elderly. There is a dearth of data from controlled studies on SUDs among the elderly and the use of pharmacologic agents for treatment, although data indicate that older adults with SUDs respond well to treatments that are specifically designed for this age group.

In their article, Cohen and colleagues discuss "Insomnia and Other Sleep Disorders in Older Adults." Sleep disruption is common in older adults and is associated with many poor health outcomes. As the worldwide population of older adults' surges, it is vital for providers to understand insomnia and other sleep disorders in this population. This article outlines age-related changes in sleep, and medical, psychiatric, environmental, and psychosocial factors that may impact sleep. It addresses evaluation of sleep symptoms and diagnosis of sleep disorders. It aims to examine the evidence for nonpharmacologic and pharmacologic treatment options for insomnia while weighing factors particularly germane to the aging adult.

In the article in this issue by Balaram and Balachandran, they discuss "Psychopharmacology in the Elderly: Why Does Age Matter?" A growing percentage of our population is aging, and a large subset meets diagnostic criteria for one or more neuropsychiatric disorders. Older adults are more likely to have several underlying medical illnesses, leading to an increased risk of polypharmacy and its associated drug-drug interactions. Commonly occurring disease states in older adults, such as bladder outlet obstruction, bowel hypomotility, and atherosclerosis, can contribute to an increased risk of adverse effects when psychotropic medications are prescribed. Physiologic changes due to aging impacts most of the pharmacokinetic processes in the body, leading to medication doses that are unintentionally subtherapeutic or supratherapeutic. Age-related physiologic changes in cardiovascular, gastric, hepatic, and renal function can also lead to changes in the pharmacokinetics of medications that can affect the absorption, distribution, accumulation, and clearance and elimination of various medications. Age-related physiologic changes further increase sensitivity of serious and potentially fatal adverse reactions, like orthostatic hypotension, cognitive impairment, arrhythmias, falls, delirium, and death. As a result, there is an ever-increasing need for continued research into the efficacy and safety of pharmacotherapy options for use in this population.

Bayer and colleagues discuss "Comorbidity and Management of Concurrent Psychiatric and Medical Disorders" in their article. Aging brings increased susceptibility to medical and psychiatric comorbidity via interrelated biologic, psychological, and social mechanisms. Mental status changes or other psychiatric symptoms occurring in older adults with medical disorders most often result from delirium, depression, or the onset of Alzheimer disease and related dementias (ADRD). Clinicians can use evidence-based tools to evaluate such symptoms, including the 4A's Test for delirium, the Saint Louis University Mental Status exam, and the Geriatric Depression Scale. Innovative models, such as collaborative care, can improve the outcome of care of older adults with medical disorders requiring treatment for depression or ADRD.

In their article, Conroy and colleagues discuss "Geriatric Psychiatry Across the Spectrum: Medical Student, Resident, and Fellow Education." The older adult population in the United States is poised to reach 83.7 million by 2050, and up to 20% will suffer from cognitive and mental illnesses. Based on these projections, general psychiatrists will provide care for an increasing number of older psychiatric patients. Enhancing learning opportunities during general medical education and residency could improve the knowledge of general psychiatrists and encourage recruitment into geriatric psychiatry. This article outlines geriatric psychiatry education in medical school, residency, and geriatric psychiatry fellowship with suggestions for recruitment into the field, along with recommendations for enhanced learning for general psychiatrists.

Louis J. Marino Jr, MD
Chief of Staff, Sheppard Pratt
6501 North Charles Street
Baltimore, MD 21204, USA

Associate Professor, Clinical
The Warren Alpert School of Medicine at Brown University
Providence, RI, USA

Distinguished Fellow, American Psychiatric Associatino

George S. Zubenko, MD, PhD
Distinguished Life Fellow, American Psychiatric Association
Fellow Emeritus, American College of Neuropsychopharmacology
Fellow (Medical Sciences), American Association for the Advancement of Science
Fellow, Royal Society of Medicine
Keystone Advanced Behavioral Healthcare, LLC
12300 Perry Highway, Suite 100
Wexford, PA 15090, USA

E-mail addresses:
louis.marino@sheppardpratt.org (L.J. Marino)
KABH12@comcast.net (G.S. Zubenko)

The Impact of Severe Acute Respiratory Syndrome-Coronavirus-2 Infection and Pandemic on Mental Health and Brain Function in the Elderly

Angela Wang, MD[a], Caitlin Lawrence, MD[a,b],*

KEYWORDS

- COVID-19 • SARS-CoV-2 • Pandemic • Elderly • Geriatric

KEY POINTS

- Direct effects of COVID-19 infection on the elderly are likely a function of illness severity, pre-existing medical and psychaitric co-morbidities, and sociocultural context.
- COVID-19 infection in the elderly had the potential to influence symptoms of anxiety, depression, insomnia, cognition, and PTSD. Non-infected individuals faced grief, isolation, and loneliness.
- The wellbeing of geriatric patients and caregivers during the COVID-19 pandemic relates to the sweeping challenges in healthcare delivery and long term care services.
- Though vulnerable to the direct and indirect effects of the COVID-19 virus, older individuals have shown resilience.

INTRODUCTION

At the precipice of its third year, the coronavirus disease (COVID-19), as a pandemic, has destabilized the well-being of individuals across the globe, and in many ways has disproportionately affected the lives of the elderly. Severe acute respiratory syndrome-coronavirus-2 (SARS-CoV-2) was first recognized in China in late 2019 as a respiratory virus with broad systemic effects and a high potential for transmissibility and lethality, spreading quickly around the globe. The World Health Organization estimates over 6 million deaths related to COVID-19 worldwide,[1] and the Centers for Disease Control and Prevention has identified nearly 975,000 deaths in the United

[a] Department of Psychiatry and Human Behavior, Warren Alpert Medical School, Brown University, Providence, RI, USA; [b] The Miriam Hospital, 164 Summit Avenue, Providence, RI 02906, USA
* Corresponding author. The Miriam Hospital, 164 Summit Avenue, Providence, RI 02906.
E-mail address: caitlin_lawrence@brown.edu

Psychiatr Clin N Am 45 (2022) 611–624
https://doi.org/10.1016/j.psc.2022.07.007
0193-953X/22/© 2022 Elsevier Inc. All rights reserved.

States,[2] over 75% in individuals over age 65. Early in the pandemic, the elderly were identified as vulnerable to severe complications and higher lethality rates. The well-being of the elderly has been a source of great concern, given the high morbidity and mortality, disruption in natural supports, sweeping social changes, and the implications of isolation precautions on these individuals. However, the elderly have long been appraised to have better emotional regulation, lower stress reactivity, and a greater sense of well-being than younger adults.[3] Understanding the overall impact of the COVID-19 pandemic on the mental health and global well-being of the elderly remains complex and requires an appraisal of the direct effects of COVID-19 infection on individuals, as well as the psychological impact of public health measures, such as lockdown protocols intended to curb the spread of the virus. At the time of the publication of this article, the preponderance of published literature examines data in the early stages of the pandemic during a time of significant fear, confusion, and uncertainty; although ongoing research is underway to better understand the later stages of the pandemic after the development of effective vaccines and loosening of social restrictions.

CASE

Mr. J is an 81-year-old man who contacted the geriatric psychiatry clinic in June of 2020 at the urging of his children. He had previously been supported in the clinic for anxiety, insomnia, and caregiver stress related to the care of his wife, who suffered from moderate dementia and had recently transitioned to a memory unit at an assisted living facility in 2019. In the wake of the pandemic, he had been unable to visit his wife for the past 3 months due to isolation protocols and an outbreak of COVID-19 in the facility. Mrs. J eventually contracted the infection and suffered from weakness, lethargy, and dehydration, requiring multiple hospitalizations and transitions to skilled nursing facilities. She had declined by this point and was minimally verbal and with a higher degree of baseline confusion, but had survived the infection. Mrs. J remained weak and unable to progress out of the nursing home, and the couple was only able to communicate during brief and infrequent phone calls, and the interactions were quite limited. Mr. J remained healthy but had been isolated at home for the past 3 months. His children limited any in-person interactions due to their wishes to avoid exposing him to the virus. Mr. J was now suffering from an increasingly depressed mood and anxiety in the wake of separation and uncertainty about his wife's trajectory. He was still able to manage his own cooking and cleaning but his children had provided assistance for grocery deliveries. He was able to connect for his telehealth visit, although troubleshooting his video conference took nearly 20 minutes, and effective communication was limited by his profound hearing impairment.

How can you understand the direct and indirect effects of the COVID-19 pandemic on Mr. J and Mrs. J?

What interventions for addressing Mr. J's symptoms were feasible at this time? How may this have changed as the pandemic progressed?

DIRECT NEUROPSYCHIATRIC EFFECTS OF CORONAVIRUS DISEASE INFECTION

Neurological symptoms of SARS-CoV-2 infection were recognized early in the pandemic and are a source of immediate concern and academic interest. Case reports of a broad spectrum of acute COVID-related neurologic events included ischemic stroke, encephalitis, epilepsy, neurodegenerative diseases, and inflammatory-mediated neurological disorders.[4] Mediators in such cases are hypothesized to include the direct neurotrophic effects of COVID-19, as well as indirect effects of hospitalization, hypoxia, use of mechanical ventilation and sedatives, systemic inflammation, and organ dysfunction.[5] Across age groups, in the early stages of the pandemic, hospitalized adults experienced high rates of COVID-related delirium[6]; and elderly patients who experienced COVID-related delirium were found to be at higher risk of subsequent longer-term cognitive decline.[7] The capability of COVID-19 to invade the blood–brain barrier, exhibit direct neurotrophic effects on the central nervous system, and directly contribute to cardiovascular and cerebrovascular disease is theorized to place the elderly population at higher longer-term risk of cognitive decline, dementia, and even motor impairment.[8]

These concerns are only a superficial summary of a larger and evolving evidence base. Neuropsychiatric effects of COVID-19 infection in the elderly are covered extensively elsewhere in this issue by Roy and Dix.

OUTCOMES OF CORONAVIRUS DISEASE INFECTION ON THE PSYCHIATRIC HEALTH OF ELDERLY INDIVIDUALS

Elderly individuals were psychologically impacted by the pandemic in different ways than their younger counterparts. In the general population, the elderly appeared more likely to express fear of COVID-19 than younger individuals, but globally had a lesser degree of psychological impact related to the pandemic and were considered to be a generally more resilient group.[9–11] However, patients who have experienced COVID-19 infections appear uniquely vulnerable to psychological symptoms compared to noninfected individuals.[12]

Research involving adult COVID-19 survivors may help guide understanding of the direct psychological effects of COVID-19 infection on the elderly, but further efforts to distinguish these two populations are necessary. One study of over 40,000 adult patients in a global health collaborative clinical research database identified a number of common psychiatric manifestations of coronavirus infection, the most prevalent being anxiety and related disorders in 4.6%, mood disorders in 3.8%, sleep disorders in 3.4%, and even suicidal ideation in 0.2%.[13] Survivors of COVID-19 are found in short-term follow-up studies to have prominent symptoms of anxiety, depression, fatigue, and insomnia,[14,15] also reflected in the persistence of elevated PHQ-9 scores 2–3 months after hospital discharge.[16] Studies up to 6-months post-infection reveal symptoms of anxiety and/or depression in 23% of participants and sleep difficulties in 26%.[17] Rates of depression in COVID-19 survivors were significantly higher than those of noninfected individuals affected by quarantine and isolation precautions.[18]

Studies specifically examining elderly COVID-19 survivors suggest that the elderly are vulnerable to psychological symptoms, especially after severe infections. In one study of hospitalized elderly COVID-19 survivors, 11.5% were identified to have clinically significant symptoms of anxiety and 46.2% to have clinically significant symptoms of depression.[19] In a small study of 69 elderly individuals 2-weeks post-hospital discharge, multiple measures of psychiatric well-being were astonishingly elevated in COVID-19 survivors when compared with age-matched healthy residents in the community—with 100% of survivors showing pathological scores in a measure of global mental health, 93.2% with symptoms of anxiety, and 86.6% with symptoms of depression.[20] A recent cohort study of 215 residents of long-term care facilities in Spain during the early stages of the pandemic identified that elderly residents, regardless of the presence or absence of initial COVID-19 infection, experienced growth rates of psychiatric symptoms at 3-month follow-up, including symptoms of depression (57.7%), anxiety (29.3%), post-traumatic stress disorder (PTSD) (19.1%), and sleep disturbance (93%); although this trend was true regardless of COVID-19 infection, those who had tested positive for COVID-19 at baseline experienced higher rates of anxiety and PTSD compared to their noninfected peers.[21]

Estimates of the incidence of PTSD symptoms in adult COVID-19 survivors are variable between studies and may be moderated by time relative to infection, the severity of infection, hospitalization, as well as the social context of the infection. One survey of clinically stable hospitalized adult COVID-19 survivors in the very early stages of the pandemic in Wuhan, China found that 96.2% had a significant degree of PTSD-spectrum symptoms on the day of hospital discharge,[22] although these would be better classified as acute stress symptoms. However, 4 months post-hospital discharge, a study of 238 COVID-19 survivors in Italy identified mild symptoms of PTSD in 25.6%, moderate symptoms in 11.3%, and severe PTSD symptoms in 5.9%.[23]

However, Horn and colleagues[24] studied patients in France with laboratory-confirmed COVID-19 infection 2 months after infection and reported that rates of clinically probable PTSD were significantly lower in patients over 60 years of age with laboratory-confirmed COVID-19 infection when compared with younger patients. Cai and colleagues[19] also found that individuals who were retired or over 60 years old had a lesser degree of PTSD symptoms associated with recent COVID-19 infection when compared with younger infected individuals and that social support appeared to be a protective factor against the development of PTSD symptoms. Some hypothesize that the elderly, despite their vulnerability to the virus, may be more able to contextualize the relative impact of the virus to other traumatic and stressful events experienced earlier in life.

Longer-term sequelae of COVID-19 infections persisting beyond 12 weeks post-infection are often referred to as "long COVID," "long-haul COVID," "chronic COVID," "post-acute COVID-19," and a variety of other terms. Ongoing research is needed to define and study this phenomenon, which according to the CDC, includes neuropsychiatric symptoms, such as fatigue, mood changes, sleep changes, and cognitive changes often described as "brain fog."[25] A systematic review by Reynaud-Charest and colleagues.[26] examined a number of studies 12+ weeks after COVID-19 infection. Their summarized interpretations suggested that data on older age as a moderator of post-COVID depressive symptoms are mixed, that severity of acute COVID-19 infection did not clearly influence persistent depressive symptoms after COVID 19 infection, and that neurocognitive impairment did not clearly influence depression. However, the presence of post-COVID depressive symptoms did significantly impair neurocognitive function.

The phenomenon of post-COVID psychosis remains a topic of discussion in case studies and case series, with little data involving the elderly, and should be interpreted in the context of the relatively high incidence of COVID-related encephalopathy and neurologic sequelae in this age group.

Not only is there concern that COVID-19 infection increased the risk of poor psychiatric outcomes in the elderly, but there is clear evidence that poor psychological health increased the risk of poor outcomes of COVID-19 infection. A Cochrane review of 21 studies, including data from 91 million individuals revealed that those with pre-existing mood disorders had higher odds of COVID-19-related hospitalizations (odds ratio 1.31) and death (odds ratio 1.51) when compared with those without pre-existing mood disorders.[27] This is hypothesized to relate to the higher rates at which individuals with mood disorders reside in congregate facilities, experience comorbid health conditions, or possibly the increased risk of inflammatory states in those with certain mood disorders.

THE INDIRECT EFFECTS OF CORONAVIRUS DISEASE ON GERIATRIC MENTAL HEALTH

Even in elderly individuals who have been fortunate enough to avoid SARS-CoV-2 infection, the indirect effects of the global pandemic on mental health and overall well-being deserve recognition. The interaction between society and the pandemic has just as much influence on geriatric mental health as the virus has on the body. The policies enacted by governing bodies around the world to combat the pandemic and their cascading effects are the most apparent indirect influences of the virus. Although jurisdictions worldwide enacted different sets of public health protocols to control viral spread, public health information campaigns, quarantine, and masking orders were relatively pervasive.

Changes in residential care, homecare, and family care

The COVID-19 pandemic had a profoundly negative impact on resources for elderly adults both in the community and in residential care settings. Indirectly, barriers to obtaining optimal supportive services placed stress on both older adults and their caregivers, contributing to suboptimal global well-being and a greater risk of poor mental health outcomes.

Adults over age 65 comprise 62.5% of adult day care utilizers, 81.9% of home health agency utilizers, 81.5% of nursing home residents, and 93.4% of residential care community residents.[28] Infections in congregate care settings spread rapidly in the early pandemic, and although case reporting was imperfect at the time and often difficult to interpret, residents in nursing home settings comprised a large proportion of COVID-19-related infections and deaths. For example, one report in May 2020 suggested that at this 2-month mark in the pandemic, 42% of deaths in the United States from COVID-19 had stemmed from the 0.6% of the population residing in a nursing home and assisted living facilities.[29] As of March 31, 2022, there were 1,011,780 confirmed cases of COVID-19 and 151,726 COVID-19-related deaths in nursing home residents in the United States.[30]

During the early waves of the pandemic, nursing homes were challenged to care for an unprecedented number of acutely ill patients in uncertain circumstances, finding it difficult to meet the needs of residents in accordance with usual quality standards. Front line nursing home staff noted multiple unique stressors impeding day-to-day care, including constraints on testing, extended use and reuse of personal protective equipment (PPE), appraising and implementing guidance from numerous regulatory agencies, increased workloads, staffing shortages, and the breakdown of organizational communication and teamwork. These practical challenges were coupled with the emotional burden of caring for residents facing isolation, severe illness, and death. Front line staffs reported increasing levels of burnout and also were demoralized by negative media coverage of nursing homes in comparison to the heroic efforts of hospital staff.[31] Nationwide, the number of nursing home staff COVID-19 infections marginally exceeded those of nursing home residents, and as of March 31, 2022, there have been 2341 staff deaths related to COVID-19 (https://data.cms.gov). Infections to the staff perpetuated burnout and drastically disrupted the continuity of care of patients in all facility settings.

For residents of congregate care settings, a paucity of PPE and vaccinations translated to extreme measures to curb the spread of coronavirus. Elderly residents were placed in "lockdown" or "isolation" arrangements, were unable to see their families, and were unable to participate in shared meals or activities. The lack of access to surveillance testing perpetuated restrictions for months.[32] The development and implementation of coronavirus vaccines drastically reduced the risk of mortality in congregate care settings and allowed for a stepwise reinstitution of community meals, stimulating group activities, and family visitation. However, COVID-19 exposures in long-term care settings continued to disrupt normal operations, including episodic lockdowns and slowing of admissions, making it difficult for patients in need of residential care to access such in a timely manner. Many families continued to experience a hesitancy to utilize congregate care environments. In these circumstances, the care of the elderly fell increasingly into the hands of family caregivers and home care agencies.

Access to adult daycare programs was uniquely disrupted during the pandemic, with a preponderance of programs closing entirely. Many elderly adults rely upon these programs for daytime structure, stimulating activities, access to basic nursing care, safe observation, and socialization. These needed services are essentially impossible to replicate in a home care environment. Closures and avoidance of adult day programs shifted responsibilities for care to in-home care and especially to informal family care internationally.[33,34] However, home care agencies were also strained during the pandemic, and often unable to match the needs of the elderly in the community. One study in Japan suggested that home care service utilization did not increase during the pandemic, despite encouragement by the Japanese government.[35] Home care service providers were financially strained and unable to grow during the pandemic, due to declines in referrals, the high cost of necessary supplies, and furloughs.[36]

Family caregivers were encouraged to implement a number of strategies to increase stimulation for recently homebound elderly individuals, including utilization of digital devices for social connection and stimulation, engaging in purposeful activities around the home, and developing a simple and predictable daily routine.[37] A small study involving spousal and adult-child caregivers of patients with dementia who received telephone support for family caregiving during the pandemic identified multiple sources of anxiety for caregivers, including the sense of isolation, increased responsibility, stress related to worsening dementia-related behaviors, restrictions of social interaction, concerns about job loss, and difficulties in adapting to COVID-19 safety recommendations.[38] Unfortunately, a sample of 897 community-dwelling older persons in the United States during the first 3 months of the pandemic identified reports of elder abuse in 21.3%, when compared with a 10% prepandemic baseline prevalence, with a sense of community appearing protective, although financial strain being associated with an increased risk of abuse.[39]

Adult day programs have slowly become more accessible when compared with the early pandemic, but are still limited and prone to unpredictable closures.

Isolation and other downstream effects of quarantine

Successful quarantining inherently and deliberately leads to isolation, the explicit goal being to seclude individuals so that person-to-person transmission is limited. Surveys around the world have reflected broad increases in the rates of loneliness, depression, and anxiety as a result of this isolation, and the risks of suicide and suicidality have risen accordingly.[40] Geriatric patients living at home often reported a decrease in physical activity, increase in fatigue and hopelessness.[41]

Although the vast majority of surveys concluded a measurable increase in loneliness, depression, and anxiety, there were a small number of studies that examined this from different perspectives that seemed somewhat more optimistic. One survey in Qatar compared older adults to the gender and age-matched controls and found that the prevalence of depressive, anxiety, and stress scores in the elderly were not significantly different.[42] However, in the quarantine group, higher depressive, anxiety, and stress scores as well as lower resilience was associated with the female gender. An Austrian survey comparing prepandemic and pandemic levels of loneliness found that although COVID-19 restrictions did result in increased levels of loneliness in the elderly, the effects were short-lived.[43] They concluded that they expect no strong negative consequences for mental health, although longitudinal studies are clearly needed.

An unintended consequence of specifically targeted quarantining policies was observed in Sweden.[44] As COVID-19 cases initially rose, the Public Health Agency in Sweden strongly advised avoiding contact with those aged 70 and above as a means to protect those deemed "weak and frail." Verbal abuse toward Swedish elderly for walking outside increased thought due to disparity in the restriction guidelines based on age.

Interventions were made in an attempt to reduce social isolation and loneliness while still being physically apart. Intuitively, direct communication through social networking websites was associated with reduced loneliness, whereas passive engagement was associated with greater loneliness.[45] Flexibility in the delivery of both loneliness and psychological interventions with cognitive behavioral therapy improved benefit. The elderly also often reported the importance of traditional communication methods, such as telephone calls. Involvement of the elderly in befriending programs demonstrated increases in self-confidence, allowing volunteers to give back to their community and benefit from social engagement. A cross-sectional study from Hong Kong showed that the elderly who continued to volunteer during the pandemic experienced fewer symptoms of depression and anxiety, suggesting that encouragement of volunteerism despite difficult circumstances can promote mental health.[46]

Grief

Owing to the higher mortality rates among the elderly, we may presume greater rates of catastrophic grief as the elderly lose friends, family, and loved ones at such an unnaturally accelerated rate. There have been countless stories of those who have died alone due to social distancing requirements, with families and friends unable to say goodbye in person. Normal bereavement processes and the social and cultural rituals they require have been universally disrupted almost without exception. The expectation was that rates of prolonged grief disorder among the elderly would naturally increase as a result.[47] A cross-sectional survey not limited to the elderly did note that where there were higher grief levels after COVID-19 bereavement than natural bereavement, grief severity was not significantly different pre- and post-pandemic. However, experiencing a loss during the pandemic elicited a more severe acute grief reaction.[48]

Personal Protective Equipment and Communication

Sensory impairments, such as reduced visual and aural acuity, are most common in the geriatric population, who are also most likely to depend on the use of hearing aids, medical equipment, and compensatory strategies, such as lip-reading to function optimally. Widespread use of PPE during the pandemic has exacerbated the existing sensory and comprehension obstacles that the elderly face when communicating with family, friends, and service providers. Barriers to effective communications can negatively impact an individual's ability to confidently maintain meaningful social connections and express his or her needs effectively, hence contributing to loneliness, anxiety, disorientation, and distress.

Providers and caregivers are encouraged to implement pragmatic strategies for mindful communication during COVID-19. This may include approaching a patient from the front, giving time for older adults to process who you are, interacting at eye level, projecting a calm attitude, using short simple sentences, and emphasizing those sentences with gestures.[49]

Reactions to public health announcement and media campaigns

Public health information campaigns have been an invaluable instrument for disseminating information about COVID-19, announcing new policies and procedures, and issuing recommendations on best practices. An information campaign that fails to convey the severity of the pandemic would induce a low level of arousal and in turn less action toward protecting oneself against the threat. At the other extreme, hyperbolic messaging may induce excessive stress and feelings of being overwhelmed, also leading to inadequate response to a threat.

Owing to the heightened morbidity and mortality in the geriatric population after COVID-19 infection, there was specific messaging in informational campaigns and in the media emphasizing the risk of the virus to the elderly,[50] which has persisted late into the pandemic.[51] Although this message was intended to protect a more vulnerable generation, this repetitive reminder throughout the pandemic also emphasized the frailty of old age and may have had the unintended consequence of framing the elderly as a burden or a liability. Although drawing on data that is accurate in that the elderly are more at risk, the framing continues to divide the young and the old. Social media carried more blatant ageist sentiments. During a time when more individuals relied on social media to feel connected during quarantine, user-generated metadata terms such as "#BoomerRemover" trended on the popular microblogging site Twitter.[52] This collected and disseminated ageist messages and became a platform for expressions of intergenerational resentment.

Racial inequality and violence

The COVID-19 death rate in the United States has disproportionately consisted of Non-Latino Black and Latino Americans,[53] which was most prominent in middle-aged adults but persisted into the 9th decade. These findings brought essential attention to sources of structural racism within these communities, noting higher rates of employment in "essential" positions, employment without paid sick leave, and living arrangements in densely populated areas or multigenerational homes.[54] Although living in close proximity to family caregivers was once a protective factor for well-being in these families, it became an unavoidable risk. Similar influences directly contributed to increased COVID-19 mortality and barriers to care among older Asian Americans.[55] The organization *Stop Asian American and Pacific Islander (AAPI) Hate* gathered data on racially motivated attacks on this group during the first year of the pandemic—of the 10,905 hate incidents reported, seniors were involved in up to 7%.[56] The National Public Radio report on the US census survey found that Asian American households were twice as likely as white households to report food scarcity at home during the pandemic due to fear of going out[57]; in some locales, community organizations were able to respond to this need with meal delivery, but it is more likely that the elderly with baseline difficulties accessing services were left to manage on their own, perpetuating fear and uncertainty.

Telehealth and access to care

In the early stages of the pandemic, the shift to telemedicine services utilizing web-based videoconferencing platforms or telephone support allowed otherwise isolated individuals to have some connection to medical and psychiatric care. Given the nature of mental health care, psychiatry was uniquely poised for a transition to telehealth services, providing access to care with minimal risk of viral exposure. Although this rapid innovation was helpful to many, the infrastructure to support this shift was not available in many lower resource countries and was often not sufficient in caring for elderly individuals with cognitive limitations.[58] Low computer literacy, poor Internet access, cognitive limitations, and sensory impairment remain barriers to the universal implementation and usefulness of telemedicine services for a substantial portion of this demographic. Although a number of modifications were made to cognitive evaluation tools to allow for virtual assessment, thorough cognitive assessments remained difficult to implement in a telehealth format. With waning in the perceived acuity of the pandemic and widespread availability of effective vaccinations and appropriate PPE, the availability of in-person care is again normalizing.

SUMMARY AND IMPLICATIONS FOR PRACTICE

Thoughtful assessment of elderly individuals will be essential for helping this cohort heal, recover, and adapt to the pandemic. This will include screening for prior COVID infection, assessing the severity of the prior infection and any short- or long-term neurocognitive effects of infection, assessing for the presence or worsening of psychiatric symptoms, appraising available social supports and changes in social engagement, identifying needs that were not met during pandemic restrictions and if these have been subsequently remedied, identifying loss and grief, and assessing for the appropriateness of in-person support versus utilization of telehealth to increase access to quality care.

Ongoing research will be essential in helping to better understand shifts in the cognitive, psychiatric, and physical health of elderly individuals during the later waves of the pandemic, and the impact of vaccination and other public health interventions on these domains.

The demand for geriatric psychiatry will grow even more precipitously in a late pandemic and post-pandemic world, and large-scale efforts to address this resource gap will be essential for the health of our communities **Boxes 1** and **2**.

Box 1
Potential components of a biopsychosocial survey of the elderly adult in the COVID-19 pandemic

- Prepandemic cognitive impairment, mental health diagnoses, and social vulnerabilities
- Before COVID-19 infection and subsequent challenges
  - Cognitive
  - Psychologic (mood, anxiety, sleep, PTSD)
  - Physical (frailty, deconditioning, falls, weight loss, worsening in medical comorbidities)
- Changes in residential circumstances
  - Hospitalizations, nursing homes, homecare, family care
- Changes in financial circumstances
  - Job loss, premature retirement, caregiver job loss
- Recent experiences of grief and loss
- Recent experiences of racial bias, social inequity, caregiver abuse or neglect
- Access to and quality of social supports and disruptions during pandemic
- Difficulty accessing resources
  - Transportation
  - Senior center, adult day services
  - Food
  - Medical appointments, medications, diagnostic studies
- Ability to participate effectively in telehealth services

Box 2
Potential resources for a transdisciplinary approach to support resilience in the elderly adult during the COVID-19 pandemic

Social work

Physical therapy

Occupational therapy

Neurology

Neuropsychology

Primary care

Geriatric psychiatry

Psychotherapy

Grief support

Geriatric care management

Caregiver support programs

Elderly protective services

Exercise programs

Reopening community services (senior centers, adult day programs, and so forth)

Volunteer opportunities

CLINICAL PEARLS

- The direct effects of severe acute respiratory syndrome coronavirus virus 2 infection in the elderly include cognitive dysfunction, anxiety, depression, insomnia, and trauma-related symptoms, although the extent to which these are disruptive is likely a function of the severity of infection, the presence of pre-existing medical and psychiatric comorbidities, and the sociocultural context of the infection.

- Sociocultural shifts during the coronavirus disease (COVID-19) pandemic generated unprecedented challenges for even noninfected individuals, relating to grief, isolation, loneliness, discrimination, and barriers to meeting basic needs.

- The COVID-19 pandemic drastically impacted the delivery of care for individuals dependent on long-term care facilities, homecare services, and adult day services, shifting the burden of care to family caregivers.

- Although older adults have experienced poor outcomes relating to cognitive health and mental health during the pandemic, they have also shown a greater degree of resilience compared to younger adults, especially in consideration of post-traumatic or acute stress symptoms.

- Providers will continue to proactively support the physical, psychological, and social health of geriatric adults affected by the COVID-19 pandemic, including screening for and treating psychiatric symptoms; assessing for cognitive dysfunction; identifying unmet day-to-day needs; promoting vaccination; and supporting a safe return to valued activities and social relationships.

- The pandemic provided the catalyst for the expansion of telehealth services in geriatric psychiatry, although in-person services remain necessary to care for the most vulnerable.

DISCLOSURE

The authors have nothing to disclose.

REFERENCES

1. WHO coronavirus (COVID-19) dashboard. Available at: https://covid19.who.int/. Accessed March 28, 2022.
2. Covid Data Tracker: United States COVID-19 cases, deaths, and laboratory testing (NAATs) by state, territory, and jurisdiction. Available at: https://covid.cdc.gov/covid-data-tracker/#cases_casesper100klast7days. Accessed March 28, 2022.
3. Lee EE, Depp C, Palmer BW, et al. High prevalence and adverse health effects of loneliness in community-dwelling adults across the lifespan. Int Psychogeriatr 2019;31(10):1447–62.
4. Achar A, Ghosh C. Covid-19-associated neurological disorders: the potential route of cns invasion and blood-brain relevance. Cells 2020;9(11):E2360.
5. Alonso-Lana S, Marquié M, Ruiz A, et al. Cognitive and neuropsychiatric manifestations of covid-19 and effects on elderly individuals with dementia. Front Aging Neurosci 2020;12:588872.
6. Mcloughlin BC, Miles A, Webb TE, et al. Functional and cognitive outcomes after COVID-19 delirium. Eur Geriatr Med 2020;11(5):857–62.
7. Liu YH, Wang YR, Wang QH, et al. Post-infection cognitive impairments in a cohort of elderly patients with COVID-19. Mol Neurodegener 2021;16(1):48.
8. de Erausquin GA, Snyder H, Carrillo M, et al. The chronic neuropsychiatric sequelae of COVID-19: The need for a prospective study of viral impact on brain functioning. Alzheimers Dement 2021;17(6):1056–65.
9. Parlapani E, Holeva V, Nikopoulou VA, et al. A review on the COVID-19-related psychological impact on older adults: vulnerable or not? Aging Clin Exp Res 2021;33(6):1729–43.
10. Palgi Y, Shrira A, Ring L, et al. The loneliness pandemic: loneliness and other concomitants of depression, anxiety and their comorbidity during the COVID-19 outbreak. J Affect Disord 2020;275:109–11.
11. Gonzalez-Sanguino C, Ausín B, Castellanos MÁ, et al. Mental health consequences during the initial stage of the 2020 Coronavirus pandemic (COVID-19) in Spain. Brain Behav Immun 2020;87:172–6.
12. Krishnamoorthy Y, Nagarajan R, Saya GK, et al. Prevalence of psychological morbidities among general population, healthcare workers and COVID-19 patients amidst the COVID-19 pandemic: A systematic review and meta-analysis. Psychiatry Res 2020;293:113382.
13. Nalleballe K, Reddy Onteddu S, Sharma R, et al. Spectrum of neuropsychiatric manifestations in COVID-19. Brain Behav Immun 2020;88:71–4.
14. Mazza MG, De Lorenzo R, Conte C, et al. Anxiety and depression in COVID-19 survivors: Role of inflammatory and clinical predictors. Brain Behav Immun 2020;89:594–600.
15. Townsend L, Dyer AH, Jones K, et al. Persistent fatigue following SARS-CoV-2 infection is common and independent of severity of initial infection. PLoS One 2020;15(11):e0240784.
16. Raman B, Cassar MP, Tunnicliffe EM, et al. Medium-term effects of SARS-CoV-2 infection on multiple vital organs, exercise capacity, cognition, quality of life and mental health, post-hospital discharge. EClinicalMedicine 2021;31:100683.

17. Huang C, Huang L, Wang Y, et al. 6-month consequences of COVID-19 in patients discharged from hospital: a cohort study. Lancet 2021;397(10270):220–32.
18. Zhang J, Lu H, Zeng H, et al. The differential psychological distress of populations affected by the COVID-19 pandemic. Brain Behav Immun 2020;87:49–50.
19. Cai X, Hu X, Ekumi IO, et al. Psychological distress and its correlates among COVID-19 survivors during early convalescence across age groups. Am J Geriatr Psychiatry 2020;28(10):1030–9.
20. Mowla A, Ghaedsharaf M, Pani A. Psychopathology in elderly covid-19 survivors and controls. J Geriatr Psychiatry Neurol 2022;35(4):467–71.
21. Cortés Zamora EB, Mas Romero M, Tabernero Sahuquillo MT, et al. Psychological and functional impact of covid-19 in long-term care facilities: the covid-a study. Am J Geriatr Psychiatry 2022;30(4):431–43.
22. Bo HX, Li W, Yang Y, et al. Posttraumatic stress symptoms and attitude toward crisis mental health services among clinically stable patients with COVID-19 in China. Psychol Med 2021;51(6):1052–3.
23. Bellan M, Soddu D, Balbo PE, et al. Respiratory and psychophysical sequelae among patients with COVID-19 four months after hospital discharge. JAMA Netw Open 2021;4(1):e2036142.
24. Horn M, Wathelet M, Amad A, et al. Prevalence and risk factors of ptsd in older survivors of covid-19 are the elderly so vulnerable? Am J Geriatr Psychiatry 2022; 30(6):740–2.
25. Post-covid conditions. Available at: https://www.cdc.gov/coronavirus/2019-ncov/long-term-effects/index.html. Accessed March 28, 2022.
26. Renaud-Charest O, Lui LMW, Eskander S, et al. Onset and frequency of depression in post-COVID-19 syndrome: A systematic review. J Psychiatr Res 2021;144: 129–37.
27. Ceban F, Nogo D, Carvalho IP, et al. Association between mood disorders and risk of covid-19 infection, hospitalization, and death: a systematic review and meta-analysis. JAMA Psychiatry 2021;78(10):1079–91.
28. Harris-Kojetin L, Sengupta M, Lendon JP, et al. Long-term care providers and services users in the United States, 2015–2016. National Center for Health Statistics. Vital Health Stat 2019;3(43).
29. Roy A. The most important coronavirus statistic: 42% of U. S. deaths are from 0.6% of the population. Forbes. Retrieved from: https://www.forbes.com/sites/theapothecary/2020/05/26/nursing-homes-assisted-living-facilities-0-6-of-the-u-s-population-43-of-u-s-covid-19-deaths/?sh=66dd2c4774cd. May 26, 2020.
30. Centers for Medicare and Medicaid Services. COVID-19 Nursing Home Data. Available at: https://data.cms.gov/covid-19/covid-19-nursing-home-data. Accessed March 28, 2022.
31. White EM, Wetle TF, Reddy A, et al. Front-line nursing home staff experiences during the covid-19 pandemic. J Am Med Dir Assoc 2021;22(1):199–203.
32. Grabowski DC, Mor V. Nursing home care in crisis in the wake of covid-19. JAMA 2020;324(1):23–4.
33. Dawson WD, Ashcroft EC, Lorenz-Dant K, et al. 2020. Mitigating the Impact of the COVID-19 Outbreak: A Review of International Measures to Support Community-Based Care.
34. Rodrigues R, Simmons C, Schmidt AE, et al. Care in times of COVID-19: the impact of the pandemic on informal caregiving in Austria. Eur J Ageing 2021; 18(2):195–205.
35. Sugawara S, Nakamura J. Long-term care at home and female work during the COVID-19 pandemic. Health Policy 2021;125(7):859–68.

36. Jones CD, Bowles KH. Emerging challenges and opportunities for home health care in the time of covid-19. J Am Med Dir Assoc 2020;21(11):1517–8.

37. Canevelli M, Bruno G, Cesari M. Providing simultaneous covid-19-sensitive and dementia-sensitive care as we transition from crisis care to ongoing care. J Am Med Dir Assoc 2020;21(7):968–9.

38. Lee J-A, Ju E, Tom C, et al. Telephone support for dementia family caregivers during the COVID-19 pandemic: Experiential differences in spouse and adult-child caregivers. Alzheimer's Dement 2021;17:e053244.

39. Chang ES, Levy BR. High prevalence of elder abuse during the covid-19 pandemic: risk and resilience factors. Am J Geriatr Psychiatry 2021;29(11): 1152–9.

40. Wand A, Zhong B, Chiu H, et al. COVID-19: the implications for suicide in older adults. Int Psychogeriatr 2020;32(10):1225–30.

41. Yurumez Korkmaz B, Gemci E, Cosarderelioglu C, et al. Attitudes of a geriatric population towards risks about COVID -19 pandemic: in the context of anxiety and depression. Psychogeriatrics 2021;21(5):730–7.

42. Ouanes S, Kumar R, Doleh E, et al. Mental Health, resilience, and religiosity in the elderly under COVID-19 quarantine in Qatar. Arch Gerontol Geriatr 2021;96: 104457.

43. Stolz E, Mayerl H, Freidl W. The impact of COVID-19 restriction measures on loneliness among older adults in Austria. Eur J Public Health 2020;31(1):44–9.

44. Skoog I. COVID-19 and mental health among older people in Sweden. Int Psychogeriatr 2020;32(10):1173–5.

45. Gorenko J, Moran C, Flynn M, et al. Social Isolation and Psychological Distress Among Older Adults Related to COVID-19: A Narrative Review of Remotely-Delivered Interventions and Recommendations. J Appl Gerontol 2020; 40(1):3–13.

46. Chan W, Chui C, Cheung J, et al. Associations between Volunteering and Mental Health during COVID-19 among Chinese Older Adults. J Gerontol Soc Work 2021;64(6):599–612.

47. Goveas J, Shear M. Grief and the COVID-19 Pandemic in Older Adults. FOCUS 2021;19(3):374–8.

48. Eisma M, Tamminga A. Grief Before and During the COVID-19 Pandemic: Multiple Group Comparisons. J Pain Symptom Manage 2020;60(6):e1–4.

49. Schlögl M, A. Jones C. Maintaining our humanity through the mask: mindful communication during COVID -19. J Am Geriatr Soc 2020;68(5):E12–3.

50. Su Z, McDonnell D, Wen J, et al. Mental health consequences of COVID-19 media coverage: the need for effective crisis communication practices. Globalization and Health 2021;17(1).

51. Leonhardt D. Covid's Risk to Older Adults. Nytimes.com. 2022. Available at: https://www.nytimes.com/2021/12/23/briefing/covids-risk-to-older-adults.html. Accessed March 20, 2022.

52. Soto-Perez-de-Celis E. Social media, ageism, and older adults during the COVID-19 pandemic. EClinicalMedicine 2020;29-30:100634.

53. Garcia M, Homan P, García C, et al. The Color of COVID-19: Structural Racism and the Disproportionate Impact of the Pandemic on Older Black and Latinx Adults. Journals Gerontol Ser B 2020;76(3):e75–80.

54. Sáenz R, Garcia MA. The disproportionate impact of covid-19 on older latino mortality: the rapidly diminishing latino paradox. J Gerontol B Psychol Sci Soc Sci 2021;76(3):e81–7.

55. Ma K, Bacong A, Kwon S, et al. The Impact of Structural Inequities on Older Asian Americans During COVID-19. Front Public Health 2021;9.

56. Stopaapihate.org. 2022 [online] Available at: https://stopaapihate.org/wp-content/uploads/2022/03/22-SAH-NationalReport-3.1.22-v9.pdf.   Accessed March 19, 2022.

57. Npr.org. More Than 9,000 Anti-Asian Incidents Have Been Reported Since The Pandemic Began. 2022. Available at: https://www.npr.org/2021/08/12/1027236499/anti-asian-hate-crimes-assaults-pandemic-incidents-aapi.   Accessed March 18, 2022.

58. Doraiswamy S, Jithesh A, Mamtani R, et al. Telehealth use in geriatrics care during the covid-19 pandemic-a scoping review and evidence synthesis. Int J Environ Res Public Health 2021;18(4):1755.

COVID-19: Brain Effects

Ebony Dix, MD*, Kamolika Roy, MD

KEYWORDS

- COVID-19 • SARS-CoV-2 • Neuropsychiatry • Long COVID • Neuroinvasion
- Neuroinflammation • Immunosenescence

KEY POINTS

- The underlying mechanisms by which severe acute respiratory syndrome coronavirus 2 affects the brain may include mechanisms related to inflammation, neuroinvasion, microvascular injury, and hypoxia.
- Brain effects may manifest as neurologic and neuropsychiatric symptoms in the acute and postacute phases of coronavirus disease, and the elderly are most vulnerable to these sequelae.
- Future research is needed to identify prevalence among other vulnerable groups, potential prognostic indicators, preventative measures, and therapeutic interventions.

INTRODUCTION

The global impact of severe acute respiratory syndrome coronavirus 2 (SARS-CoV-2), the novel coronavirus responsible for the COVID-19 pandemic, has been particularly profound and enduring for the elderly. Since the beginning of the pandemic, organizations, such as the World Health Organization (WHO) and the Centers for Disease Control and Prevention (CDC), have warned about the elevated risk of severe illness and death due to COVID-19 in the aging population.[1,2] The elderly, defined by the WHO as age 60 and older and by the CDC as age 65 and older, have the highest rates of morbidity and mortality following infection from COVID-19.[2,3] The elderly are most vulnerable to adverse outcomes due to medical comorbidities and age-related physiological changes in the brain and immune system.[4–7] Although the focus here will be on the neurobiological mechanisms and increased viral susceptibility with age, it is important to recognize the influence that racial, ethnic, cultural, and socioeconomic disparities may have on worsening health outcomes in this age demographic.[8–10]

As ongoing research continues to unfold, there is growing evidence that COVID-19 causes pathological changes in the brain and alters cellular functioning via neuroinvasion, inflammation, microvascular injury, and hypoxia.[4,11–15] Emerging data reveal that

Department of Psychiatry, Yale School of Medicine, 300 George St., Suite 901, New Haven, CT 06511, USA
* Corresponding author.
E-mail address: ebony.dix@yale.edu

Psychiatr Clin N Am 45 (2022) 625–637
https://doi.org/10.1016/j.psc.2022.07.009
0193-953X/22/© 2022 Elsevier Inc. All rights reserved.

neuropsychiatric manifestations of COVID-19 occur in both the acute and postacute phases of illness, and for some these symptoms persist for weeks to months after recovering from COVID-19 illness.[15,16]

This reality has broader implications for the pathogenicity of the SARS-CoV-2 virus when considering the increased vulnerability of the brain with aging, especially in those with premorbid cognitive impairment and dementia.[6–8,17–20] Epidemiological studies illustrate that acute manifestations of neurological and neuropsychiatric disease occur in up to 80% of hospitalized cases.[13,21] In milder cases of COVID-19, these symptoms occur in the absence of typical respiratory symptoms[4,5,13] In the elderly, postmortem histological and radiological studies reveal morphological changes in brain structure in addition to evidence of neurovascular injury within the central nervous system (CNS), suggesting potentially irreversible damage to the brain.[5,15,22–28]

Here, we summarize the most updated evidence underlying the proposed neuropathological and immunological processes by which COVID-19 impacts the brain. Given the rapid growth of knowledge being disseminated on this topic, we recognize that some of the proposed mechanisms have still to be fully elucidated and understood. First, we give a brief overview of some of the known characteristics of SARS-CoV-2 that have been proposed to facilitate inflammation and neuronal injury leading to direct brain effects. We discuss the mechanisms by which the elderly may be more vulnerable to these potentially indelible effects. Then, we highlight the neurological and neuropsychiatric symptoms that have been reported in the literature and review the potential brain regions that may be implicated in some of the long-term sequelae. We conclude with a summary of the current recommendations for the prevention and treatment of COVID-19 in addition to a discussion of areas for future research and development.

Proposed Mechanisms: What Is it and How Does it Infect the Brain?

Similar to other strains of coronaviruses, such as the Middle East Respiratory Syndrome and Severe Acute Respiratory Syndrome-Coronavirus, SARS-CoV-2 is hypothesized to enter the CNS by a variety of mechanisms.[11,15,29] The former viruses have demonstrated an ability to enter the brain stem and replicate, however, to date, there is insufficient data to support the ability of SARS-CoV-2 to do the same.[6,30]

SARS-CoV-2 is part of a family of enveloped, positive-sense, single stranded RNA viruses with viral spike (S) protein that bind to host cell entry receptors, namely, angiotensin converting-enzyme 2 (ACE2).[4,13–15] It has been proposed that ACE2 is the key transmembrane receptor on host endothelial cells to which the S-protein binds.[4,11,31] The fusion of cell and viral membranes is further enabled by cleavage of the S-protein attached to ACE2 by the host cell transmembrane protease, serine 2, allowing the virus to enter cells.[4,11,31]

Although the ACE2 receptor has a wide distribution of systemic tissue expression, there is a high ACE2 receptor density in the cerebral microcirculation.[15] The high burden of neurological and neuropsychiatric symptoms observed in COVID-19 suggests a particular viral tropism favoring entry through the CNS or the peripheral nervous system.[14,30] SARS-CoV-2 has high affinity for ACE2 receptors in cerebral microcirculation and it has been proposed that the virus may travel via nerves innervating the respiratory tract, a primary site for replication.[11,15] Specifically, CNS invasion of cranial nerves via axonal transport, such as on olfactory nerve endings, have been described in the literature.[14,15,32] Alternatively, SARS-CoV-2 may bind ACE2 receptors on olfactory epithelial cells and enter via tight junctions. In addition to viral tropism, it has been suggested that SARS-CoV-2 is capable of hematogenous spread, enabling disruption of the blood–brain barrier (BBB) or the blood–cerebrospinal fluid barrier (B-CSFB).[11,15] Regardless of the precise route of viral cell entry, the resulting endothelial cell damage triggers a neuroinflammatory response that is thought to be responsible for microvascular injury, leading to stroke, vasculitis, organ failure, and effects on the brain.[9,11,15,33,34] The influx of inflammatory mediators known as "cytokine storm" and upregulation of the coagulation cascade are implicated in the activation of microglial cells.[4,7,11,14,15] There is subsequent neurotransmission dysfunction and neuronal cell loss resulting in neurological and neuropsychiatric symptoms.[4,7,11,14,15,35] **Fig. 1** is a schematic illustration summarizing the proposed mechanisms.[4,11,13,14,33-35]

Mechanisms of severe acute respiratory syndrome coronavirus 2 neuroinvasion[4,11,13,14,33-35]

1. *Infection*: SARS-CoV-2 respiratory droplets enter sustentacular cells of the olfactory epithelium. Hematogenous transmission is via ACE2 receptor binding to vascular endothelium. Endothelial damage triggers microthrombus formation, increased von Willebrand factor (vWF), fibrin deposition, and platelet activation. Systemic infection leads to oxidative stress, hypoxia, and a hyperinflammatory state.

2. *Neuronal transmission:* Neuronal injury and infection trigger recruitment and activation of immune cells, including glial cells, astrocytes, macrophages, and T-lymphocytes. SARS-CoV-2 neuroinvasion causes neuroinflammation by way of cytokine storm [production and release of tumor necrosis factor-alpha, interleukin-6 (IL-6), IL-10, and IL-1β] that directly induces microglial activation and indirectly triggers coagulation cascade (which leads to further microglial activation).

3. *CNS pathophysiology:* Microglial activation leads to increased kynurenine production, which increases quinolinic acid (increases glutamate and upregulates N-methyl-D-aspartate receptors) and depletes neurotransmitters (serotonin, dopamine, and norepinephrine). Altered neurotransmission and excitotoxicity by increased glutamate and hypoxic injury contribute to neuronal dysfunction and cell death. Demyelination (due to oligodendroglial cell death) leads to neuronal excitotoxicity, hypoxia, and synaptic alterations. Cytokine storm leads to neuroinflammation, increased vascular permeability, dysfunction of BBB and BCSFB, and subsequent neurodegeneration. Coagulation cascade and elevation of vWF lead to thrombotic events. Hypercoagulation increases D-dimer, fibrinogen and thrombus formation.

Neurologic and Neuropsychiatric Manifestations

During the COVID-19 pandemic, the nomenclature has emerged to identify neurologic and neuropsychiatric symptoms as they related to specific periods of time during COVID-19 illness. Acute symptoms have been reported in the literature to last up to approximately 4 weeks and include delirium, encephalitis, stroke, and psychiatric disorders.[13,20,33,34,36,37] For the purposes of this article, the term *postacute* will refer to chronic or long-term neuropsychiatric symptoms lasting any time beyond 4 weeks after acute infection. In the published literature to date, many refer to long-term neuropsychiatric symptoms that continue for 12 weeks or more, after one has recovered from COVID-19 illness.[38] The term "long COVID" is gaining recognition as a way to identify some of the symptoms that have lasting effects on individuals long after their recovery from acute infection.[15,38,39] There is little understood as of the writing of this article the exact etiologies or risk factors for this condition, especially as symptom development does not correlate with the severity of COVID-19 illness.[15,38,39] The constellation of symptoms associated with long COVID is also sometimes referred

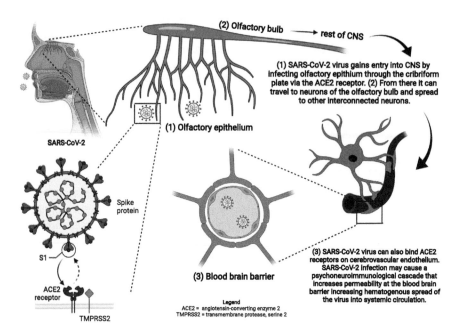

Fig. 1. A schematic summarizing the proposed mechanisms. ACE2, angiotensin converting-enzyme 2; TMPRSS2, transmembrane protease, serine 2. (Created with BioRender.com.)

to as the postacute sequelae of COVID-19 (PASC) and may be used interchangeably in this discussion.[40–42] The phenomenon of long COVID is unique in that it appears to represent a protracted course of neurologic and neuropsychiatric sequelae across all age groups. Long COVID has been reported to include a wide range of symptoms, including dyspnea, fatigue, sleep disturbances, and neuropsychiatric symptoms, such as headache, memory loss, concentration, and changes in mood.[2,13–16,38,40] One proposed mechanism for the lasting brain effects after recovering from acute illness is that SARS-CoV-2 remains dormant in neurons and the delayed effect of neuroinflammation leads to demyelination and neurodegeneration.[43]

Due to the increasing prevalence of these symptoms and their impact on daily functioning, there is still much to be learned and understood about what causes these sequelae and how they may be prevented or reversed.[32,33,38,40] Broadly, acute effects of viral infection can include acute stroke, neuromuscular dysfunction, demyelinating disorders, encephalopathy, confusion, emotional disturbances, and psychosis. Acute neurological events in individuals over age 50 most commonly include cerebrovascular events followed by anosmia/hyposmia, and hypogeusia, and those aged 65 and older more commonly present with confusion and stroke symptoms.[22,44–46]

Delirium is often multifactorial in nature and in the elderly, it may be the first acute presenting symptom of COVID-19, creating a diagnostic challenge and possible delays in care. There is some evidence that suggests individuals who experienced delirium during their acute illness were likely to be affected by PASC.[41]

Some of the postacute neuropsychiatric sequelae commonly noted in the literature include depression, anxiety, cognitive difficulties, including memory impairment, inattention, executive dysfunction, concentration difficulty as well as headache.[3,22,43] In

Table 1
Neurologic and neuropsychiatric manifestations

	Acute Coronavirus Disease	Postacute Coronavirus Disease
Neurologic symptoms	Anosmia, hyposmia Hypogeusia, dysgeusia Encephalitis Stroke Neuromuscular dysfunction Demyelinating disorders Acute encephalopathy[a]	Anosmia Encephalopathy Encephalitis Stroke Headache Neurodegeneration Demyelination Neuropathy

Neuropsychiatric symptoms	Psychiatric Disorders
	  Mood disorders
	  Catatonia
	  Anxiety
	  Insomnia
	  Psychosis
	Neurocognitive Disorders
	  Delirium[a]
	  Major/minor neurocognitive
	    disorder
		Psychiatric Disorders
		  Mood disorders
		  Anxiety
		  Insomnia
		  Psychosis
		  Post-traumatic stress disorder
		Neurocognitive disorders
		  Cognitive impairment—memory
		    deficits, inattention,
		    executive dysfunction

[a] Interchangeable per updated nomenclature guidelines in Slooter et al.

those hospitalized due to COVID-19, anxiety, depression, sleep impairment, and post-traumatic disorder comprised the longstanding PASC **Table 1**.[33]

Neurological symptoms

- CNS effects: anosmia, ageusia, stroke—hemorrhagic and ischemic, CNS vasculitis, acute inflammation of brain, spinal cord, meninges leading to encephalitis or encephalopathy.[47]
- PNS effects: neuromuscular disorders, such as Guillain–Barré syndrome, Miller Fisher variant, Bell's palsy, and other demyelinating neuropathies, epilepsy (direct versus indirect cause; secondary to cytokine storm). Nonspecific neurological manifestations include headache, fatigue, and myalgias.[30,47]

Neuropsychiatric symptoms

- Neuropsychiatric symptoms secondary to excitotoxicity and hypoxic injury and differ depending on the Brodmann area involved.
- Acute psychiatric symptoms include depression, anxiety, insomnia, memory impairment, psychosis, and delirium/encephalopathy (acute confusion and agitation).[47] Many of these may persist as late neuropsychiatric sequelae, including depression, suicidal behavior, anxiety, psychosis, seizures, insomnia, fatigue, post-traumatic stress, attention deficits, memory impairment and irritability, encephalitis lethargica (caused by 1918 influenza pandemic), and limbic encephalitis.[34]

What does neuroimaging research reveal about brain changes due to coronavirus disease?. The literature concerning the effects of the SARS-CoV-2 virus on the brain continues to expand and there is no exception when reviewing neuroimaging research available on this topic. As we enter the third year of the pandemic, the data collected and analyzed have also evolved. Earlier radiological studies aimed at characterizing abnormal neuroimaging findings on MRI and computed tomography (CT) scans in COVID-19-infected individuals, including cerebral microhemorrhages, acute spontaneous intracranial hemorrhage, acute and subacute infarcts, and encephalitis or encephalopathy.[48] Subsequent systematic reviews with meta-analysis of MRI, PET, and CT studies have revealed specific brain regions that may be structurally and functionally affected in COVID-19, such as the olfactory cortex extending to prefrontal and limbic regions.[28]

Many of these neuroimaging studies have suggested COVID-19 brain-related pathologies in the elderly (age > 60 years) in the brain stem and frontotemporal regions, including cerebrovascular injury, hypoperfusion, evidence of inflammation, and cellular damage along white matter tracts.[22,44–46] Such investigations have identified risk factors that contribute to the severity of COVID-19 illness, such as pre-existing neurological illness, psychiatric illness, sleep disturbance, immunosenescence, and hyperinflammatory states with age. However, investigations thus far have been unable to isolate the direct impact of pathogenicity of SARS-CoV-2 infection in the brain.

More recently, the UK Biobank COVID-19 re-imaging case-control study has been the first and largest of its kind to elucidate statistically significant longitudinal changes in the brain due to SARS-CoV-2 infection by comparing neuroimaging scans from affected individuals both pre- and post- COVID-19 infection.[5] Early evidence from this study suggests a greater reduction in global brain size, the possibility of the left cerebral hemisphere being more strongly associated with SARS-CoV2 infection, and longitudinal limbic olfactory brain changes involving functionally connected regions of anterior cingulate cortex, orbitofrontal cortex, amygdala, hippocampus, and parahippocampal gyrus.[5]

Primary brain regions demonstrating altered structure or function on neuroimaging include the olfactory cortex and subsequent projection areas, such as the orbitofrontal cortex, amygdala, insula, entorhinal cortex, and hippocampus.[28] Neuroimaging findings involving brain regions implicated in COVID-19 infection are summarized in **Table 2**, which summarizes findings derived from a review of case series, cohort studies, and systematic reviews.[13]

Considerations for coronavirus disease in persons with dementia. Early during the COVID-19 pandemic, the elderly were identified as the most vulnerable population to SARS-CoV-2 infection due to the increased burden of pre-existing medical comorbidities, frailty, and age-related immune system dysfunction known as immunosenescence.[4,49] Further review of literature on effects of COVID-19 in the elderly reveals an atypical course of symptom presentation, which may include no fever or low-grade fever and the absence of common respiratory symptoms, such as dyspnea and cough, which may lead to delayed diagnosis of COVID-19 in the geriatric population.[3]

Atypical symptom presentation is also common in persons with dementia who contract COVID-19 and may manifest as exacerbation of cognitive decline, impairment in activities of daily living, or worsening behavioral and psychological symptoms of dementia (BPSD). However, delirium is commonly the first presenting symptom in persons with dementia with acute SARS-CoV-2 infection.[34] Using a validated measurement tool for detecting delirium, such as the Confusion Assessment Method, is recommended but there is currently no existing equivalent tool for detecting long COVID or post-acute sequelae of COVID (PASC).

Underlying cognitive impairment is known to be associated with higher rates of delirium due to medical illness and it is well known that delirium may be protracted in individuals with dementia. Therefore, not surprisingly, persons with mild cognitive

Table 2
Neuroimaging findings on the brain regions implicated in severe acute respiratory syndrome coronavirus 2

	Brain Regions	Imaging Findings	Studies	Imaging Modalities	Study Design
Cortical regions	Anterior cingulate cortex (PFC)	Impairments in connectivity and signal intensity (functional MRI), fluorodeoxyglucose hypometabolism (PET)	Najt et al,[28] 2021	MRI, PET, computed tomography	Systematic review and meta-analysis
		Greater reduction in gray matter thickness and tissue-contrast (MRI)	Douaud et al,[5] 2022	MRI, functional MRI	Case control cohort study
	Orbitofrontal cortex prefrontal cortex (PFC)	Fluorodeoxyglucose hypometabolism (PET)	Najt et al,[28] 2021	MRI, PET, computed tomography	Systematic review and meta-analysis
	Olfactory cortex (limbic)	Greater changes in markers of tissue damage (functional MRI)	Douaud et al,[5] 2022	MRI, functional MRI	Case control cohort study
		Altered cortical volume, thickness and hypometabolism	Najt et al,[28] 2021	MRI, PET, computed tomography	Systematic review and meta-analysis
	Insula (limbic)	Low gray matter volume/reduced cortical thickness (MRI)	Douaud et al,[5] 2022	MRI, functional MRI	Case control cohort study
		Fluorodeoxyglucose hypometabolism (PET)	Najt et al,[28] 2021	MRI, PET, computed tomography	Systematic review and meta-analysis
	Superior temporal gyrus (limbic)	Reduced cortical thickness	Najt et al,[28] 2021	MRI, PET, computed tomography	Systematic review and meta-analysis
	Parahippocampal gyrus (limbic)	Greater reduction in gray matter thickness and tissue contrast	Douaud et al,[5] 2022	MRI, functional MRI	Case control cohort study
		Fluorodeoxyglucose hypometabolism (PET)	Najt et al,[28] 2021	MRI, PET, computed tomography	Systematic review and meta-analysis

(continued on next page)

Table 2
(continued)

Brain Regions		Imaging Findings	Studies	Imaging Modalities	Study Design
Subcortical regions	Entorhinal cortex	Greater changes in markers of tissue damage (functional MRI)	Douaud et al,[5] 2022	MRI, functional MRI	Case control cohort study
	Thalamus	Fluorodeoxyglucose hypometabolism (PET)	Najt et al,[28] 2021	MRI, PET, computed tomography	Systematic review and meta-analysis
	Amygdala (limbic)	Fluorodeoxyglucose hypometabolism (PET)	Najt et al,[28] 2021	MRI, PET, computed tomography	Systematic review and meta-analysis
	Hippocampus (limbic)	Low gray matter volume/ reduced cortical thickness, decreased cerebral blood flow (MRI)	Najt et al,[28] 2021	MRI, PET, computed tomography	Systematic review and meta-analysis
	Corpus callosum	Increased diffusivity indicating tissue damage, white matter abnormalities due to microhemorrhage (MRI)	Najt et al,[28] 2021	MRI, PET, computed tomography	Systematic review and meta-analysis
	Brain stem	White matter and volume abnormalities due to microhemorrhage (MRI) FDG hypometabolism (PET)	Najt et al,[28] 2021	MRI, PET, computed tomography	Systematic review and meta-analysis

mpairment or dementia who contract the SARS-CoV-2 virus are at greater risk of severe illness and are more vulnerable to long-term neuropsychiatric sequelae.[22,34,44–46] Specifically, persons with dementia due to underlying neurodegenerative diseases such as Alzheimer's disease or Parkinson's disease, may experience an exacerbation of preexisting BPSD due to COVID-19; therefore, monitoring for changes can be essential for early detection of acute infection. Symptom overlap with BPSD and long-term neuropsychiatric sequelae, such as agitation, apathy, and aberrant motor activity, presents a challenge to those caring for persons with dementia.[30]

Treatment Recommendations

There is currently limited published data to support the use of any specific agent for the treatment or prevention of neuropsychiatric sequelae of COVID-19. Multiple national organizations, such as the WHO and CDC, and The National Institutes of Health, have highly recommended vaccination for all eligible elderly to prevent and reduce the risk of severe illness.[2] As of the time of this writing, The National Institutes of Health COVID-19 Treatment Guidelines Panel continues to update its Web site regarding the therapeutic management of hospitalized and nonhospitalized adults. The guidance on clinical management of COVID-19 inpatients changes rapidly as we gain a better understanding of the virus. Current knowledge about SARS-CoV-2 has enabled the use of therapeutic agents, such as antivirals, like remdesivir, and immunomodulators, such as corticosteroids and monoclonal antibodies.[31,49] There is some hope that an improved understanding of the mechanisms of these drugs will inspire future research and development of immunotherapeutic agents that can potentially mitigate the acute and postacute brain effects of COVID-19. In the absence of a more novel approach, for now, the use of pre-existing evidence-based treatments and standards of care will continue to be employed for treating the neurologic and neuropsychiatric symptoms that emerge from COVID-19. For the treatment of delirium, there is no clinical consensus; however, there is a growing body of data that supports the efficacy of using low-dose neuroleptics and alpha-adrenergic blockers for managing symptoms.[2,50,51] However, the ever-present challenge in the pharmacological treatment of delirium in the elderly with COVID-19 will be to carefully avoid adverse events due to drug interactions, or medical contraindications and to weigh the risks versus benefits of those agents known to be potentially harmful in the elderly.[52]

SUMMARY

In conclusion, the long-term effects of COVID-19 on the brain have left an indelible imprint on the global community. Whether acute or postacute, brain effects have impacted individuals across all age groups, irrespective of the severity of COVID-19 illness. The knowledge regarding the neuropathology of the virus suggests that by way of neuroinvasion and hyperinflammation, neurologic and neuropsychiatric symptoms may emerge and persist for an extended period, well after one has recovered from COVID-19. Data also suggest that a major risk factor for lasting brain effects is age, and the neuropsychiatric sequelae present a greater burden on the elderly, especially those with premorbid cognitive impairment.[8,18,20,33,46] Detecting delirium or changes in baseline behavior in the elderly may be an early key finding in the acute phase of illness, given the propensity for atypical COVID-19 presentations in this age group.

As the current understanding of the neurochemical and immunological processes underlying the brain effects of COVID-19 continues to evolve, lessons learned up to this point during the pandemic will undoubtedly pave the way for future research and innovation. By applying the current knowledge about how the brain and immune system respond to acute COVID-19 infection, we will hopefully soon identify other risk factors and prognostic indicators in a variety of other populations. Areas of need for further research include epidemiological studies that identify the true prevalence and incidence of long COVID across the life span and any potentially irreversible sequelae. It will be equally important to ensure such studies not only look at all age groups and at people who have been both vaccinated and unvaccinated, but also at individuals of diverse backgrounds and geographical regions. Given the existing health care disparities related to race, ethnicity, and socioeconomic status, the pandemic presents an opportunity for a critical look at how biopsychosocial factors might influence the development of future vaccines and immunotherapies.[2]

CLINICS CARE POINTS

- Severe acute respiratory syndrome coronavirus 2 infection causes acute and postacute neurologic and neuropsychiatric symptoms, some of which persist for weeks to months, and is known as long coronavirus disease (COVID-19) or post-acute sequelae of COVID-19 (PASC).
- Neuropathological mechanisms have been hypothesized to trigger neuroinflammation, causing downstream effects on neurotransmitters and leading to a myriad of symptoms.
- Increased vulnerability of the brain with aging places the elderly, especially those with cognitive impairment, at an increased risk for neuropsychiatric sequelae from COVID-19.
- People with dementia may have atypical presentations of COVID-19, which lead to delays in diagnosis and increased risk of severe illness and death.
- People with dementia are at an increased risk of persistent postacute neuropsychiatric sequelae, which may be difficult to differentiate from worsening dementia.
- In caring for people with dementia, monitoring for changes in baseline mentation (delirium) or worsening of pre-existing behavioral disturbances may be the earliest way to detect acute COVID-19 infection.
- A better understanding of the mechanisms by which COVID-19 affects the brain will pave the way for future research and the development of potential preventative and therapeutic approaches.

DISCLOSURE

The authors have nothing to disclose.

REFERENCES

1. De Pue S, Gillebert C, Dierckx E, et al. The impact of the COVID-19 pandemic on wellbeing and cognitive functioning of older adults. Sci Rep 2021;11(1):4636.
2. World Health Organization. Regional Office for the Western P. Guidance on COVID-19 for the care of older people and people living in long-term care facilities, other non-acute care facilities and home care. 2020. Available at: http://iris. wpro.who.int/handle/10665.1/14500. Accessed April 1, 2020.
3. Bansod S, Ahirwar AK, Sakarde A, et al. COVID-19 and geriatric population: from pathophysiology to clinical perspectives. Horm Mol Biol Clin Investig 2021;42(1): 87–98.
4. Chen Y, Klein SL, Garibaldi BT, et al. Aging in COVID-19: Vulnerability, immunity and intervention. Ageing Res Rev 2021;65:101205.

5. Douaud G, Lee S, Alfaro-Almagro F, et al. SARS-CoV-2 is associated with changes in brain structure in UK Biobank. Nature 2022. https://doi.org/10.1038/s41586-022-04569-5.

6. Mainali S, Darsie ME. Neurologic and neuroscientific evidence in aged COVID-19 Patients. Front Aging Neurosci 2021;13:648662.

7. Perrotta F, Corbi G, Mazzeo G, et al. COVID-19 and the elderly: insights into pathogenesis and clinical decision-making. Aging Clin Exp Res 2020;32(8): 1599–608. https://doi.org/10.1007/s40520-020-01631-y.

8. Hampshire A, Trender W, Chamberlain SR, et al. Cognitive deficits in people who have recovered from COVID-19. EClinicalMedicine 2021;39:101044.

9. Wang Z, Zheutlin A, Kao YH, et al. Hospitalised COVID-19 patients of the Mount Sinai Health System: a retrospective observational study using the electronic medical records. BMJ Open 2020;10(10):e040441.

10. Willey B, Mimmack K, Gagliardi G, et al. Racial and socioeconomic status differences in stress, posttraumatic growth, and mental health in an older adult cohort during the COVID-19 pandemic. EClinicalMedicine 2022;45:101343.

11. Boldrini M, Canoll PD, Klein RS. How COVID-19 Affects the Brain. JAMA Psychiatry 2021;78(6):682–3.

12. Butler M, Bano F, Calcia M, et al. Clozapine prescribing in COVID-19 positive medical inpatients: a case series. Ther Adv Psychopharmacol 2020;10. https://doi.org/10.1177/2045125320959560.

13. Han Y, Yuan K, Wang Z, et al. Neuropsychiatric manifestations of COVID-19, potential neurotropic mechanisms, and therapeutic interventions. Transl Psychiatry 2021;11(1):499. https://doi.org/10.1038/s41398-021-01629-8.

14. Johansson A, Mohamed MS, Moulin TC, et al. Neurological manifestations of COVID-19: a comprehensive literature review and discussion of mechanisms. J Neuroimmunol 2021;358:577658.

15. Bauer L, Laksono BM, de Vrij FMS, et al. The neuroinvasiveness, neurotropism, and neurovirulence of SARS-CoV-2. Trends Neurosci 2022. https://doi.org/10.1016/j.tins.2022.02.006.

16. Taquet M, Geddes JR, Ilusain M, et al. 6-month neurological and psychiatric out comes in 236 379 survivors of COVID-19: a retrospective cohort study using electronic health records. Lancet Psychiatry 2021;8(5):416–27.

17. Aghagoli G, Gallo Marin B, Katchur NJ, et al. Neurological involvement in COVID-19 and potential mechanisms: a review. Neurocrit Care 2021;34(3):1062–71.

18. Lebrasseur A, Fortin-Bédard N, Lettre J, et al. Impact of the COVID-19 pandemic on older adults: rapid review. JMIR Aging 2021;4(2):e26474.

19. Nersesjan V, Fonsmark L, Christensen RHB, et al. Neuropsychiatric and cognitive outcomes in patients 6 months after COVID-19 requiring hospitalization compared with matched control patients hospitalized for Non-COVID-19 illness. JAMA Psychiatry 2022. https://doi.org/10.1001/jamapsychiatry.2022.0284.

20. Simonetti A, Pais C, Jones M, et al. Neuropsychiatric symptoms in elderly with dementia during COVID-19 Pandemic: definition, treatment, and future directions. Front Psychiatry 2020;11:579842.

21. Chou SH, Beghi E, Helbok R, et al. Global incidence of neurological manifestations among patients hospitalized With COVID-19-A report for the GCS-NeuroCOVID consortium and the ENERGY consortium. JAMA Netw Open 2021;4(5):e2112131.

22. Frontera JA, Yang D, Lewis A, et al. A prospective study of long-term outcomes among hospitalized COVID-19 patients with and without neurological complications. J Neurol Sci 2021;426:117486.

23. Huang C, Huang L, Wang Y, et al. 6-month consequences of COVID-19 in patients discharged from hospital: a cohort study. Lancet 2021;397(10270):220–32.
24. Kremer S, Gerevini S, Ramos A, et al. Neuroimaging in patients with COVID-19: a neuroradiology expert group consensus. Eur Radiol 2022;1–10. https://doi.org/10.1007/s00330-021-08499-0.
25. Kremer S, Lersy F, Anheim M, et al. Neurologic and neuroimaging findings in patients with COVID-19: A retrospective multicenter study. Neurology 2020;95(13):e1868–82.
26. Kremer S, Lersy F, de Sèze J, et al. Brain MRI findings in severe COVID-19: a retrospective observational study. Radiology 2020;297(2):E242–51.
27. Lersy F, Benotmane I, Helms J, et al. Cerebrospinal fluid features in patients with coronavirus disease 2019 and neurological manifestations: correlation with brain magnetic resonance imaging findings in 58 patients. J Infect Dis 2021;223(4):600–9. https://doi.org/10.1093/infdis/jiaa745.
28. Najt P, Richards HL, Fortune DG. Brain imaging in patients with COVID-19: a systematic review. Brain Behav Immun Health 2021;16:100290.
29. Roy D, Ghosh R, Dubey S, et al. Neurological and neuropsychiatric impacts of COVID-19 pandemic. Can J Neurol Sci 2021;48(1):9–24.
30. Manolis TA, Apostolopoulos EJ, Manolis AA, et al. COVID-19 infection: a neuropsychiatric perspective. J Neuropsychiatry Clin Neurosci Fall 2021;33(4):266–79.
31. V'Kovski P, Kratzel A, Steiner S, et al. Coronavirus biology and replication: implications for SARS-CoV-2. Nat Rev Microbiol 2021;19(3):155–70.
32. Qin Y, Wu J, Chen T, et al. Long-term microstructure and cerebral blood flow changes in patients recovered from COVID-19 without neurological manifestations. J Clin Invest 2021;131(8). https://doi.org/10.1172/jci147329.
33. Alonso-Lana S, Marquié M, Ruiz A, et al. Cognitive and neuropsychiatric manifestations of COVID-19 and effects on elderly individuals with dementia. Front Aging Neurosci 2020;12:588872.
34. Nakamura ZM, Nash RP, Laughon SL, et al. Neuropsychiatric complications of COVID-19. Curr Psychiatry Rep 2021;23(5):25.
35. Sawlani V, Scotton S, Nader K, et al. COVID-19-related intracranial imaging findings: a large single-centre experience. Clin Radiol 2021;76(2):108–16.
36. Burchill E, Rogers JP, Needham D, et al. Neuropsychiatric disorders and COVID-19. Lancet Psychiatry 2021;8(7):564–5.
37. Rogers JP, Chesney E, Oliver D, et al. Psychiatric and neuropsychiatric syndromes and COVID-19 - Authors' reply. Lancet Psychiatry 2020;7(8):664–5.
38. National Institute for Health and Care Excellence (NICE). COVID-19 rapid guideline: managing the long-term effects of COVID-19. [NG191]. https://www.nice.org.uk/guidance/ng191.
39. Butler M, Cross B, Hafeez D, et al. Emerging knowledge of the neurobiology of COVID-19. Psychiatr Clin North Am 2022;45(1):29–43.
40. The Lancet N. Long COVID: understanding the neurological effects. Lancet Neurol 2021;20(4):247.
41. Cray HV, Vahia IV. Two years of COVID-19: understanding impact and implications for the mental health of older adults. Am J Geriatr Psychiatry 2022;30(4):444–7.
42. Tabacof L, Tosto-Mancuso J, Wood J, et al. Post-acute COVID-19 syndrome negatively impacts physical function, cognitive function, health-related quality of life, and participation. Am J Phys Med Rehabil 2022;101(1):48–52.
43. Kumar S, Veldhuis A, Malhotra T. Neuropsychiatric and cognitive sequelae of COVID-19. Front Psychol 2021;12:577529.

44. Frontera JA, Melmed K, Fang T, et al. Toxic metabolic encephalopathy in hospitalized patients with COVID-19. Neurocrit Care 2021;35(3):693–706.
45. Beghi E, Giussani G, Westenberg E, et al. Acute and post-acute neurological manifestations of COVID-19: present findings, critical appraisal, and future directions. J Neurol 2021;1–10. https://doi.org/10.1007/s00415-021-10848-4.
46. Frontera JA, Wisniewski T. Editorial: neurological and neuroscientific evidence in aged COVID-19 patients. Front Aging Neurosci 2021;13:774318.
47. Slooter AJC, Otte WM, Devlin JW, et al. Updated nomenclature of delirium and acute encephalopathy: statement of ten Societies. Intensive Care Med 2020; 46(5):1020–2.
48. Choi Y, Lee MK. Neuroimaging findings of brain MRI and CT in patients with COVID-19: a systematic review and meta-analysis. Eur J Radiol 2020;133: 109393.
49. van Eijk LE, Binkhorst M, Bourgonje AR, et al. COVID-19: immunopathology, pathophysiological mechanisms, and treatment options. J Pathol 2021;254(4): 307–31.
50. Baller EB, Hogan CS, Fusunyan MA, et al. Neurocovid: pharmacological recommendations for delirium associated with COVID-19. Psychosomatics 2020;61(6): 585–96.
51. Velásquez-Tirado JD, Trzepacz PT, Franco JG. Etiologies of delirium in consecutive COVID-19 inpatients and the relationship between severity of delirium and COVID-19 in a prospective study with follow-up. J Neuropsychiatry Clin Neurosci 2021;33(3):210–8.
52. American geriatrics society 2019 updated AGS beers criteria® for potentially inappropriate medication use in older adults. J Am Geriatr Soc 2019;67(4): 674–94.

Cognitive Impairment in Older Adults
Epidemiology, Diagnosis, and Treatment

Nicolás Pérez Palmer, MD[a,*], Barbara Trejo Ortega, MD[a],
Pallavi Joshi, DO, MA[b,c]

KEYWORDS

- Neurocognitive disorder • Dementia • Mild cognitive impairment (MCI)
- Assessment • Treatment • Alzheimer's disease • Vascular dementia
- Frontotemporal dementia

KEY POINTS

- Cognitive impairment and dementia affect millions of older adults leading to significant distress and disability that often goes unrecognized.
- A systematic assessment composed of the clinical interview, physical examination, objective cognitive examination tool, neuroimaging, and laboratory workup can effectively identify these disorders.
- Management consists of a combination of non-pharmacological and pharmacological treatments focused on reducing the burden of the disease on patients and their caregivers by delaying the progression of cognitive decline and loss of functionality, and treating neuropsychiatric symptoms when present.

INTRODUCTION

With an increasingly aging population, health care providers will treat a higher number of patients with cognitive impairment. Identifying cognitive impairment and intervening early can improve the quality of life of our patients and their caregivers. However, without a systematic approach to the diagnosis and management of cognitive impairment, the spectrum of disorders can be challenging to differentiate. This article aims to provide a guideline for health care providers to diagnose and treat cognitive impairment in older adults.

[a] Department of Psychiatry, Yale School of Medicine, 300 George Street, Suite 901, New Haven, CT 06511, USA; [b] Banner Alzheimer's Institute, 901 East Willeta Street, Phoenix, AZ 85006, USA; [c] Department of Psychiatry, University of Arizona College of Medicine-Phoenix, 475 North 5th, Phoenix, AZ 85004, USA
* Corresponding author.
E-mail address: nicolas.perez-palmer@yale.edu

Psychiatr Clin N Am 45 (2022) 639–661
https://doi.org/10.1016/j.psc.2022.07.010
0193-953X/22/© 2022 Elsevier Inc. All rights reserved.

Mild cognitive impairment (MCI), also termed mild neurocognitive disorder (mNCD), signifies a loss of cognitive abilities or skills that does not cause significant functional impairment, differentiating it from dementia.[1] Cognitive impairment can be further qualified as amnestic or non-amnestic, with memory being the main affected domain in the former, whereas other domains such as executive function are primarily affected in the latter.[1] Other domains potentially affected in neurocognitive disorders include learning, language, social cognition, attention, and visuospatial function. MCI has a prevalence of approximately 6% in ages 60–64 and increases to approximately 25% in those age 80–84.[2]

Dementia or major neurocognitive disorder (MNCD) is characterized by a loss of cognitive abilities in multiple domains that leads to significant functional impairment. Approximately 5%–10% of people with MCI progress to dementia annually.[3] The underlying etiologies of dementia include Alzheimer's disease (AD), vascular dementia (VaD), mixed (Alzheimer's and vascular), frontotemporal dementia (FTD), dementia with Lewy bodies (DLB), and cognitive impairment associated with Parkinson's disease, prion disease, Huntington's disease, and others.

The burden of dementia is significant on individual, community, national, and global levels. It is projected as the fifth leading cause of death in the world and the third leading cause of death in the United States in 2017.[4,5] The amount of unpaid care from over 11 million caregivers in 1 year is estimated at 15.3 billion hours[6] and contributes to emotional, physical, and financial strain, which becomes more poignant in minority communities.[7] Compared with those without dementia, patients with dementia, aged 65 or older, account for 3 and 23 times the amount of payments per-person services through Medicare and Medicaid, respectively. The total cost of care for people with dementia is over $300 billion annually in the United States, with over $1 trillion spent on a global scale.[6]

EPIDEMIOLOGY

On a global scale, dementia affects between 6 and 50 million people, with the increasing estimates in more recent publications (either due to an increase in prevalence or increase in diagnosis).[8,9] The global prevalence of dementia appears to double every 5 years for patients between the ages of 50 and 80 years. In the United States, the prevalence of dementia in people aged 68 or older is 15%, and increases with age, doubling every 5 years after the age of 65.[10] Although prevalence worldwide has increased, the age-specific incidence for dementia may be decreasing. Mitigation of risk factors such as education level and access to health care could be playing a role in this decrease.[9]

AD affects over 5 million people in the United States and accounts for approximately 60% of dementia cases.[6,8–10] FTD accounts for the majority of cases among individuals under 65 years of age, and makes up between 1.7% and 7% of total dementia cases.[11–13] DLB ranges from 3% to over 20% of cases. Of patients with Parkinson's disease, approximately 20%–30% develop Parkinson's disease dementia (PDD) that represents approximately 3% of all dementia cases.[11,14–18] Estimates have varied significantly between studies, hinting at the challenges of diagnosing and studying the epidemiology of these conditions.

Given the population-level impact of MCI and dementia, identifying and mitigating risk factors such as older age, female gender, and racial or ethnic identity is crucial. Of note, the impact of sex is possibly confounded by longer life expectancy in women but could be due to a variety of factors.[19] Chronic conditions such as depression, hypertension, heart failure, diabetes mellitus, stroke, obstructive sleep apnea, hearing loss, and head injury have also been implicated.[8–10,20] These are impacted by diet, physical activity, smoking, and alcohol consumption, which elevate risk as well.

Higher level of education appears to be protective, although its impact on cognitive reserve possibly differs according to race—one study found that higher education level was protective of white matter hyperdensity as a measure of brain integrity for White patients but not for Black or Latino patients. Notably, higher social activity or contact, independent of education level, seems to also be protective.[21] The opportunity to mitigate risk factors in general cannot be understated. These alone have been reported to account for up to 40% of cases globally.[9]

CLINICAL ASSESSMENT

The initial clinical evaluation for an older adult presenting with cognitive impairment should consist of a thorough clinical interview with a collateral historian including a functional assessment; a physical examination including a focused neurological examination and mental status examination; a brief objective cognitive examination tool; selected laboratory tests to assess for reversible causes of cognitive impairment; and structural brain imaging.

Interview

Evaluation of cognitive impairment requires thorough history taking from the patient and collateral, usually a close family member or friend. Collateral information is key since some patients may have trouble recalling pertinent details or lack insight into their condition. In cases of more advanced cognitive impairment, a collateral informant may be the only source of information available.

When assessing the patient's subjective cognitive complaints, it is imperative to characterize the nature, magnitude, and course to create a detailed timeline of the change. The assessment includes functionality, which can be key in determining the etiology.[22] **Table 1** summarizes some of the representative symptoms for each domain.

A thorough functional assessment of the patient's instrumental activities of daily living (iADLs) and basic activities of daily living (ADLs) is imperative when differentiating between mNCD and MNCD and in characterizing the severity of MNCD. IADLs are activities that allow for independent living in the community such as shopping, food preparation, housekeeping, and finances; ADLs encompass basic activities such as feeding, dressing, bathing, toileting, and ambulation. Some of the available instruments include the Functional Assessment Staging Tool (FAST Scale), The Lawton Instrumental Activities of Daily Living (IADL) Scale, and Katz Index of Independence in ADL.

The interview should also focus on the history of medical conditions that could affect cognition (**Table 2**).

A family history of hereditable conditions associated with cognitive impairment is salient when considering heritable dementias such as early-onset AD (EOAD) and Huntington's. Family history should encompass all psychiatric disorders given the heterogeneity in the presentation of neurocognitive disorders.

Objective Cognitive Measures

A bedside standardized cognitive test is essential. The most commonly used are the Montreal Cognitive Assessment (MoCA), mini-mental status examination (MMSE), and St Louis University Mental Status Examination (SLUMS). The MoCA is more sensitive and comprehensive in identifying cognitive decline compared with the MMSE.[23] Both the SLUMS and MoCA have been found to be more sensitive than the MMSE in detecting MCI.[3] Several comparative studies have found the MoCA and SLUMS to

Table 1
Cognitive domains and representative symptoms[22,123,124]

Cognitive Domain	Clinical Question
Attention and concentration	• Does the patient walk into a room and forget why? • Does the patient have difficulty focusing on a task like reading or watching TV?
Executive function	• Does the patient have difficulties with tasks that have several steps like preparing a full meal, planning a trip, or making a schedule? • Does the patient struggle to solve problems when compared with before? • Can the patient handle appliances or gadgets like the TV remote control as well as before?
Memory and Learning	• Does the patient have difficulty recalling recent events? • Does the patient ask repetitive question? • Does the patient repeat comments or stories repetitively? • Does the patient have difficulty remembering pertinent details of recent major events like a family wedding, holiday or trip?
Language	• Does the patient have word finding difficulties or talks around words? • Does the patient have difficulty understanding the gist of conversations? • Does the patient have difficulty communicating their thoughts? • Does the patient speak in short or grammatically incorrect sentences?
Visuospatial abilities	• Does the patient have difficulty finding their way while driving? Finding the way back to the table after going to the restroom in a restaurant? • Does the patient have trouble telling time on an analog clock?
Social cognition	• Can the patient behave appropriately in social situations? Interactions with other people? • Has the patient become impulsive or reckless?

Table 2
Medical conditions associated with cognitive impairment

Interview: Identifying Other Factors Affecting Cognition	
Vascular risk factors	Diabetes, hypertension, and hypercholesterolemia
Nutritional deficiencies	Vitamin B1, vitamin B12, and folic acid
Metabolic disease	Hypothyroidism, chronic uremia, hepatic disease, and hypoglycemia
Infectious disease	Syphilis and HIV
Existing brain conditions	Parkinson's disease, traumatic brain injury, stroke, normal pressure hydrocephalus
Primary psychiatric conditions	Mood disorders, anxiety disorders, attention deficit hyperactivity disorder, posttraumatic stress disorder, psychotic disorders, substance use disorders, and obstructive sleep apnea
Medications	Anticholinergics, benzodiazepines, and analgesics

be similarly effective at detecting MCI and dementia.[24,25] In contrast to the MMSE and MoCA, which are both copyrighted, the SLUMS can be used without incurring a charge. Formal neuropsychological testing, which provides a comprehensive profile of each cognitive domain, may be pursued if the cognitive deficits are either border-line, or for highly educated and highly functioning patients.[3,26]

Physical/Neurological Examination

The physical/neurological examination, including a mental status examination, is partic-ularly useful to assess the cause of cognitive impairment. Vital signs can identify hyper-tension or dysrhythmias, both risk factors for cerebrovascular disease and orthostatic hypotension often seen in synucleinopathies such as DLB and PDD. Assessing speech quality, speed, pitch, and articulation for the presence of dysarthria is key, as it can point to different neurocognitive disorders like PDD, multiple system atrophy (MSA), progres-sive supranuclear palsy (PSP), and FTD. The use of "smell cards" can help identify ol-factory dysfunction, seen in early DLB and AD.[27,28] The presence of focal neurological signs could suggest an underlying VaD. These include aphasia, apraxia, hemineglect, motor weakness, hyperreflexia, visual field deficits, and somatosensory loss. Assessing for involuntary movements like resting tremor (seen in PDD and DLB), postural tremor (seen in DLB), myoclonus (seen in prion disease or late in the course of AD), and chorea (seen in Huntington's disease) is beneficial. Gait disturbances can be seen in several of the dementias: a parkinsonian gait (seen in PDD and DLB) is char-acterized by short strides, reduced arm swing, *en bloc* turn, and stooped posture; limb circumduction (seen in VaD) is associated with hemiparetic gait; a frontal gait pattern (seen in normal pressure hydrocephalus [NPH]) consists of "magnetic gait," poor gait initiation, and a widened base. Identification of any of these neurological signs often warrants referral to a specialist for further assessment.[22]

Blood tests and imaging

Blood tests are useful in excluding some reversible comorbidities. These include vitamin B12, folate, thyroid-stimulating hormone (TSH), calcium, glucose, complete blood cell count, renal, liver function, rapid plasma reagin test, and HIV.[29,30] Structural neuroimaging is useful in identifying potentially treatable causes of cognitive impair-ment such as a resectable tumor or NPH, and in identifying specific patterns observed in different neurocognitive disorders. Although computed tomography (CT) and mag-netic resonance imaging (MRI) are both routinely used to rule out reversible causes of cognitive impairment, MRI is more sensitive in identifying vascular pathology and pat-terns seen in other dementia etiologies such as AD.[31]

DETERMINING THE ETIOLOGY

Once the reversible causes of cognitive impairment have been ruled out and the diag-nosis of dementia is confirmed, then we can work up the etiology. Although in most cases a definite etiology can only be done postmortem, establishing a probable etiol-ogy is necessary to choose an appropriate treatment regimen.

Major neurocognitive disorder due to Alzheimer's disease

Clinical features
Current models conceptualize the progression of the disease in three phases: preclin-ical AD, MCI due to AD, and dementia due to AD.[32] Current clinical guidelines recom-mend against screening for AD in asymptomatic individuals. The diagnosis of MCI due to AD and dementia due to AD is based on the Diagnostic and Statistical Manual of

Mental Disorders, fifth edition (DSM-5) criteria, and the National Institute on Aging and Alzheimer's Association (NIA-AA) guidelines.[30,33]

The typical presentation of AD consists of slowly progressive memory decline with an insidious onset. However, less common non-amnestic forms of AD have a different presentation. Early on, individuals with AD typically present with impairment in memory and thinking that often manifests as subtle forgetfulness, occasional repetition of stories, and, of special importance, difficulty recalling the details of recent events. In contrast, memories of the distant past, immediate recollection of a recently learned address or phone number, or memory for vocabulary or concepts are not commonly affected early in the disease. As the disease progresses other cognitive domains become affected with executive function and problem-solving typically the first to deteriorate. Although the extent and rate of progression varies between individuals, a framework of stages (mild, moderate, and severe) based on the extent of functional impairment present is applied. In the milder stages, individuals are relatively independent in many iADLs but require assistance in more complex activities (eg, filing taxes). Functioning in ADLs is preserved in the milder stages. Moderate stages are characterized by difficulties in some of the ADLs, whereas individuals in the severe stage consistently need assistance with almost all ADLs.

Neuropsychiatric symptoms (NPS) are common in AD and up to 97% of individuals with AD will show at least one NPS throughout the course of the disease.[34] NPS often prompt evaluation, and their presence is associated with a more rapid functional decline and shorter survival time.[35] The most common NPS, in order of prevalence, are apathy, depression, aggression/agitation, anxiety, sleep disturbances, irritability, appetite disorder, aberrant motor behavior (eg, pacing), and delusions.[35] These symptoms can be present at any stage of the disease, including MCI, and are often comorbid with each other.

Biomarkers

Biomarkers for AD are widely used in research with well-defined guidelines, but their use in clinical settings is not established.[36] The proposed *AT(N)* classification system is also useful to quantify the disease process. Biomarkers are grouped based on the pathological process each measure (*A*: β amyloid deposition; *T*: tau deposition; *N*: neurodegeneration) and are encompassed by imaging (MRI and positron emission tomography [PET]) and fluid-based (cerebrospinal fluid [CSF] and plasma) biomarkers.

Imaging

MRI can show brain atrophy, PET can show β-amyloid or tau deposition, and fluorodeoxyglucose (FDG) PET hypometabolism can be a biomarker for neurodegeneration.[31] Structural MRI is the only widely available neuroimaging modality. Amyloid PET has limited clinical utilization outside of research; however, no health insurance reimburses its high cost other than the Veterans Health Administration where it is only approved when ordered by a dementia expert.

Fluid biomarkers

Fluid-based (CSF and plasma) biomarkers are less commonly used outside of research. These include low CSF Aβ42 and low CSF Aβ42/AB40 ratio which point to β-amyloid (Aβ) deposition. Biomarkers for Tau deposition and neurodegeneration include CSF phosphorylated tau (P-tau), and elevated CSF total tau, respectively.

Biomarker evidence of neurodegeneration is the least specific finding in AD but is useful in staging the disease. Of note, individuals with cognitive impairment concomitant with biomarker evidence of Aβ deposition and a second biomarker (T or N) have a significantly increased rate of cognitive decline compared with individuals who have neither or only Aβ deposition.[36] Several blood biomarkers are being developed for

Aβ deposition, tau deposition, and neurodegeneration. Although these blood biomarkers are currently used for research purposes, there is great promise that they will eventually be used in clinical practice given their similar efficiency in detecting biomarker abnormalities when compared with more expensive imaging biomarkers and more invasive CSF biomarkers.

When do we test for biomarkers in the clinic?
There are several proposed clinical guidelines for the use of biomarkers in AD: American Academy of Neurology (AAN), NIA-AA, and Appropriate Use Criteria for Amyloid PET Imaging. The NIA-AA guidelines recommend that MRI, PET, or CSF biomarkers be used as optional clinical tools for use where available and when deemed appropriate by the clinician to enhance the certainty of AD pathophysiology.[29] Amyloid PET can be appropriately used by a dementia expert as a single piece of information to support or oppose a clinical diagnosis of AD in a patient in whom cognitive impairment has been objectively verified, in whom there is substantial uncertainty as to the underlying pathology, and for whom greater diagnostic certainty would change management.[37] The AAN practice guidelines suggest that there is not enough evidence to support or refute PET or CSF biomarkers.[2] Overall, AD biomarkers are used as a supportive diagnostic tool in clinical practice only when the clinician deems their use will change the management, not as a routine test.

Genetics
There are several genes that increase the risk of developing AD but genetic testing is almost exclusively used in research. The apolipoprotein E (APOE) e4 gene is the most impactful in increasing the risk of developing the late-onset form of the disease (LOAD), which accounts for approximately 95% of cases. There are three forms of the APOE gene: e2, e3, and e4. An estimated 47% of individuals with a single copy of e4 and 91% of those with two copies of e4 will develop AD.[38] Having the e2 form may decrease the risk of developing AD. Approximately 25% of AD cases are estimated to be familial.

Approximately 5%–10% of cases of AD develop before age 65, a manifestation known as EOAD. The familial form of EOAD develops from rare autosomal dominant mutations in the genes for amyloid precursor protein (APP), presenilin 1 protein (PSEN1), or presenilin 2 protein (PSEN2), which carry a penetrance of 95%–100%.[39]

Genetic testing for LOAD is not routinely recommended given its limited clinical utility. Tests for genes associated with EOAD are useful in symptomatic individuals with a diagnosis of EOAD, individuals with a family history of dementia with one or more cases of EOAD, and individuals with a relative affected by a known mutation of APP, PSEN1, or PSEN2.[40] There are significant ethical aspects to genetic testing in AD, especially when pursued in asymptomatic individuals. Formal genetic counseling is key in cases where this avenue is being explored.[41]

Major vascular neurocognitive disorder

Clinical features
Vascular cognitive impairment does not have a discrete clinical presentation given the heterogeneity of the underlying vascular pathophysiology. Moreover, vascular cognitive impairment rarely occurs in isolation, with pure VD only accounting for 10% of cases.[42] The clinical presentation and neuropsychological pattern varies depending on the underlying vascular insult. Nevertheless, individuals with vascular cognitive impairment tend to perform worse on tests for executive function compared with those for memory and have impairments in processing speed.[43]

Per the DSM-V criteria, cerebrovascular disease is the dominant, if not exclusive, pathology accounting for complex attention and frontal-executive cognitive decline.[33]

Neuroimaging is key for the proper diagnosis of vascular cognitive impairment. Although CT and MRI can both be used, MRI more accurately identifies parenchymal injury attributable to cerebrovascular disease Vascular pathologies can be divided into different categorical etiologies.[44]

Large vessel/embolic disease includes poststroke or multi-infarct cognitive impairment which usually manifests as abrupt cognitive deficits that start after the stroke and plateau after weeks or months. A "stepwise" worsening in cognition can be observed if another stroke were to ensue. Physical examination signs include aphasia, apraxia, hemineglect, lateralized weakness, visual field loss, or somatosensory loss.

Small vessel disease associated with hypertensive arteriopathy includes white matter hyperintensities which are common findings on MRI and increase with age. Thus, their mere presence is not indicative of cognitive impairment.[44] When the white matter disease is significant enough, executive and/or memory impairment manifests insidiously without overt neurological signs. Apathy, psychomotor slowing, gait disturbances, and subtle speech changes can also develop.[45–47] In contrast with poststroke cognitive impairment, cognitive impairment associated with small vessel ischemic disease often slowly progresses on par with white matter hyperintensity progression.

Small vessel disease related to cerebral amyloid angiopathy is caused by pathological deposition of β-amyloid that leads to an increased risk of small vessel hemorrhage. It can cause recurrent, transient ischemic attack-like symptoms that are often described as moving through contiguous body regions.[48] Although cerebral amyloid angiopathy often co-occurs with AD, in it by itself can lead to impaired episodic memory and decreased perceptual speed.[49] Close attention to any clinical history of strokes or transient ischemic attacks is paramount when approaching an individual with suspected vascular cognitive impairment. Individuals should also be assessed for cerebrovascular risk factors such as diabetes mellitus, hypertension, hyperlipidemia, atrial fibrillation, or smoking. Focal neurological signs can often be identified with a physical examination. Brain MRI serves to confirm the presence of cerebrovascular disease and helps determine the underlying mechanism.

Genetics

There are several genetic disorders that can lead to vascular cognitive impairment. Cerebral autosomal dominant arteriopathy with subcortical infarct and leukoencephalopathy (CADASIL) is a hereditary small vessel disease that commonly leads to cognitive impairment in cognitive speed, executive function, and attention[50] It is caused by mutations in the NOTCH3 gene and is often associated to strokes and migraine headaches. Cerebral autosomal recessive arteriopathy with subcortical infarcts and leukoencephalopathy (CARASIL) is also a hereditary VD syndrome that leads to ischemic small vessel disease. It occurs because of mutations in the *HTRA1* gene.[51] A familial form of cerebral amyloid angiopathy has been linked with mutations in the APP, ITM2B, and CST3 genes.[52–54]

Major frontotemporal neurocognitive disorder

FTD, a heterogenous group of neurogenerative diseases that predominantly target the frontal and temporal lobes, can be classified into two syndromes—behavioral variant FTD (bvFTD) and Primary Progressive Aphasia (PPA). PPA is further classified into semantic variant PPA (svPPA), nonfluent variant PPA (nfvPPA), and logopenic variant PPA (lvPPA).

Behavioral variant frontotemporal dementia

bvFTD is characterized by an early onset and progressive decline in executive function and interpersonal skills with a loss of emotional and social awareness. The diagnostic criteria for bvFTD focus on changes in behavior and personality accompanied by executive dysfunction with relative sparing of memory and visuospatial domains. Behavioral symptoms include social disinhibition, apathy, abulia, loss of empathy, emotional blunting, perseverative, stereotyped or compulsive behavior, hyperorality, and dietary changes.[33,55] It is important to especially assess for features of motor neuron disease and/or extrapyramidal deficits, as Parkinsonian features are seen in 25%–80% of FTD cases with the most common symptoms being bradykinesia, parkinsonian gait, and rigidity.[56–58] International consensus on diagnostic criteria for bvFTD requires imaging results consistent with frontal and/or anterior temporal atrophy on MRI or CT, or frontal and/or anterior temporal hypoperfusion or hypometabolism on PET or single-photon emission computerized tomography (SPECT) for a diagnosis of probable bvFTD.[55]

Primary progressive aphasia

Semantic Variant PPA is characterized by a progressive decline in semantic memory which mediates knowledge of words, objects, and concepts. This often manifests as forgetting the names of objects and familiar words (spoken or in writing). Circumlocutions (the use of many words when fewer will do) and imprecise approximations of words (ie, "tiger" becomes "cat," that becomes "animal," and eventually "thing.") are common. Imaging supported diagnosis of svPPA is similar to bvFTD[59]

nfvPPA is a later onset disease compared with the other variants, with prominent deficits in speech production characterized by effortful, hesitant, and poorly constructed speech.[58] Speech errors can manifest as defective syllable selection, phonological errors, binary reversals (ie, confusion between yes and no or his and her), and/or grammatical errors. Supportive neuroimaging findings include evidence of predominant left posterior frontoinsular atrophy on MRI or left posterior frontoinsular hypoperfusion or hypometabolism on SPECT or PET.[59]

lvPPA is characterized by a difficulty in the retrieval of correct words, names, or numbers as well as difficulty with repetition and comprehension of sentences.[60] In contrast to svPPA and nfvPPA, the primary underlying etiology of lvPPA is AD pathology rather than FTD-like pathology.[61] Typical neuroimaging findings include atrophy of the temporoparietal region with more predominance in the left hemisphere and less prominent atrophy in the medial parietal lobe.[62] Amyloid PET is also often positive in lvPPA.[63]

Lastly, several causative mutations have been linked to FTD with an autosomal dominant mode of inheritance found in up to 27% of all FTD cases. A strong familial inheritance has been identified in bvFTD, with between 30% and 50% of individuals with the condition having a positive family history and a clear autosomal dominant inheritance pattern seen in 10%–15% of cases.[64–67]

Major neurocognitive disorder with Lewy bodies and major neurocognitive disorder due to Parkinson's disease

DLB and PDD are both synucleinopathies that share many clinical features. Both disorders affect cognition and behavior like other neurocognitive disorders, but DLB and PDD share a significant motor and autonomic component not typically found in other dementias. DLB and PDD are considered to be two presentations of the same disease spectrum and are clinically indistinguishable in the severe stages of the disease. The main difference between DLB and PDD lies in the temporality of motor symptoms onset; motor symptoms develop before cognitive symptoms in PDD, whereas motor symptoms either happen at the same time or follow cognitive symptoms within a year in DLB.[68]

In 2017, the diagnostic criteria for DLB were updated to include biomarker evidence of the disease as part of the criteria[69] The disorder has an insidious onset and gradual progression with deficits in attention, executive function, and visuospatial

---

Box 1
DLB core and supportive clinical features and indicative and supportive biomarkers[69]

Clinical features and biomarkers of dementia with Lewy bodies
  Core clinical features
    Fluctuating cognition with pronounced variations in attention and alertness.
    Recurrent visual hallucinations.
    Rapid eye movement (REM) sleep behavior disorder.
    One or more spontaneous cardinal features of parkinsonism: bradykinesia, rest tremor, or rigidity
  Supportive clinical features
    Severe sensitivity to antipsychotic agents; postural instability; repeated falls; syncope or other transient episodes of unresponsiveness; severe autonomic dysfunction, for example, constipation, orthostatic hypotension, urinary incontinence; hypersomnia; hyposmia; hallucinations in other modalities; systematized delusion; apathy, anxiety, and depression.
  Indicative biomarkers
    Reduced dopamine transporter uptake in basal ganglia on SPECT or PET scan.
    Abnormal 123iodine-MIBG myocardial scintigraphy.
    Polysomnographic confirmation of REM sleep without atonia.
  Supportive Biomarkers
    Relative preservation of medial temporal lobe structures on computed tomography/MRI scan,
    Generalized low uptake on SPECT/PET scan with reduced occipital activity.
    Prominent posterior slow-wave activity on electroencephalogram (EEG) with periodic fluctuations in the pre-alpha/theta range.

Probable DLB is diagnosed if two or more core clinical features of DLB are present with or without the presence of indicative biomarkers, or if only one core clinical feature is present with one or more indicative biomarkers. Possible DLB is diagnosed if one core clinical feature is present with no indicative biomarker evidence, or if one or more indicative biomarkers are present with no core clinical features.

---

function.[69,70] **Box 1** lists the core and supportive clinical features, and the indicative and supportive biomarkers.

The fluctuations seen in DLB are typically delirium-like characterized by waxing and waning episodes of behavioral changes, incoherent speech, variable attention, or altered consciousness involving staring or "zoning-out." A useful way to assess these fluctuations is to ask about daytime drowsiness, lethargy, staring into space, or episodic disorganized speech.[69] Visual hallucinations, which occur in up to 80% of individuals with DLB, are usually well-formed and detailed often featuring people, children, or animals. Insight into hallucinations is often preserved and there is little emotional content related to the hallucinations[70] Although the use of scales is recommended when assessing for RBD, it is very likely in cases where dreams have a chasing or attacking theme, and if the individual or bed partner has sustained injuries from limb movements.[71]

MANAGEMENT

The management of nonreversible neurocognitive disorders focuses on reducing the burden of the disease on patients and their caregivers by delaying the progression of cognitive decline and loss of functionality and treating NPS when present. Both non-pharmacological and pharmacological treatments are available and are often used in conjunction. Treatment should be tailored based on the etiology and severity of the neurocognitive disorder; nevertheless, some non-pharmacological treatments are often useful in any kind of neurocognitive disorder.

Table 2 lists common reversible causes of neurocognitive impairment. The goal is to treat the underlying cause.

Mild Neurocognitive Disorder/Mild Cognitive Impairment

Pharmacological treatment

Up until 2021, there were no US Food and Drug Administration (FDA) approved pharmacological treatments for MCI. Aduhelm (aducanumab), a novel amyloid β-directed monoclonal antibody, received accelerated FDA approval for early AD (MCI and mild dementia due to AD). However, questions regarding its efficacy and safety remain as well as concerns regarding its cost ($28,000 per year for the drug; the average annual cost of treatment estimated to exceed $75,000).[72] It is currently scheduled to start its phase 4 confirmatory trials in May 2022 which are projected to conclude by 2026. The Center for Medicare & Medicaid Services (CMS) recently published its decision to cover monoclonal antibodies directed against amyloid for the treatment of AD only for participants of clinical trials. Cholinesterase inhibitors (ChEIs) have limited evidence in improving cognition and delaying the progression to dementia.[73–75] Evidence on vitamins, antioxidants, and supplements has been inconclusive.[76–80]

Non-pharmacological treatment

Management of MCI focuses on lifestyle modifications to try to slow the progression of cognitive impairment. Diet, exercise, and cognitive stimulation have shown to be effective, albeit modestly, in this regard. Consistent adherence to the "Mediterranean diet" has been shown to slow the decline in cognitive impairment.[81]

The Mediterranean-DASH diet Intervention for Neurological Delay (MIND) diet, a hybrid of the Dietary Approaches to Stop Hypertension (DASH) and the Mediterranean diet, was developed specifically for dementia prevention by emphasizing the dietary components and servings linked to neuroprotection.[82] The MIND diet has been shown to be superior to other plant diets, including the Mediterranean diet, in decreasing the risk of some types of neurocognitive disorder, slowing the progression of cognitive decline, and has even been found to improve cognition.[82–84] **Table 3** gives a brief overview of the MIND diet. When possible, consulting a nutritionist to assist with implementing the MIND diet may prove helpful.

Physical exercise has been shown to slow cognitive decline and promote independent functioning in MCI and in dementia.[85] Although most of the studies have focused on aerobic exercise as an intervention, the ideal type or amount of physical activity needed to maximize its benefits on cognition is still not well understood.

Cognitively stimulating leisure activities may also be effective in delaying cognitive decline.[86–88] Although most of the studies have been conducted on older adults with normal cognition, implementing them is usually a worthwhile endeavor, given the minimal to non-existent risk of these activities. Examples are board games, crossword puzzles, word-seek-and-find puzzles, jigsaw puzzles, playing card games, playing an instrument, and socialization[3] Cognitive stimulation therapy (CST) is a brief psychological treatment for people with mild-to-moderate dementia that has proven to be effective in improving cognitive function and quality of life.[89] Similar programs have recently been trialed for individuals with MCI which suggest they may also delay cognitive decline in this population.[90]

Major Neurocognitive Disorders/Dementias

Pharmacological treatment

Aducanumab is the only disease-modifying therapy approved only for MNCD due to AD. There are another five FDA-approved pharmacologic treatments in the United

Table 3
Brief overview of the Mediterranean-DASH diet Intervention for Neurological Delay (MIND) diet[82]

Food Group	Servings
Whole grains	3 or more per day
Green leafy vegetables	2 or more per day
Other vegetables	1 or more per day
Berries	2 or more per week
Fish	1 or more per week
Poultry	2 or more per week
Beans	3 or more per week
Nuts	5 or more per week
Olive oil	Primary oil
Butter, margarine	Less than 1 tablespoon per day
Red meats and products	Less than 4 per week
Fast and fried food	Less than 1 per week
Cheese	Less than 1 per week
Pastries and sweets	Less than 5 per week
Wine	Less than 1 glass per week

States for MNCD due to AD: three ChEIs (donepezil, rivastigmine, and galantamine), an N-methyl-D-aspartate receptor antagonist (memantine), and a fixed-dose combination drug of memantine and donepezil.[91]

ChEIs have evidence for slowing the progression of cognitive decline as well as modestly improving ADL.[92] Although the efficacy among ChEI is similar, their adverse effect profile varies. **Table 4** lists the different ChEIs and their indications, dosage titration, and common adverse effects. Overall, a slow titration over 4 to 8 weeks is recommended. If adverse effects arise the medication can be discontinued and a different one in the same class can be trialed. Memantine is FDA approved for moderate-to-severe AD and it can be used as monotherapy or in combination with a ChEI. There is evidence that combination therapy with a ChEI and memantine is more beneficial for cognitive and functional function in a patient with moderate-to-severe AD when compared with monotherapy with a ChEI.[93,94] Common practice is to start with a ChEI in the mild stages of AD and then to add memantine once the disease progresses to the moderate stages. Memantine monotherapy is usually reserved for individuals who cannot tolerate a ChEI.[8]

ChEIs and memantine have little benefit in vascular disease. Donepezil has shown slight benefit in cognition in a recent meta-analysis, but without evidence for clinical significance.[95,96] Management focuses on optimally managing vascular risk factors.[97]

ChEIs and memantine are not recommended in any of the FTD subtypes and may cause behavioral symptoms to worsen.[98,99]

Both rivastigmine and donepezil have robust evidence for cognitive benefit in LBD and PPD. Galantamine has substantially less evidence.[100–102] Donepezil and rivastigmine also have evidence for improving NPS including hallucinations.[100] Memantine has mixed evidence for efficacy in cognition and NPS in DLB and PPD.[102] The common approach is to use either donepezil or rivastigmine as first line and to only use galantamine if these are not tolerated. Management of the motor symptoms, sleep disturbances, and autonomic dysfunction should be coordinated with specialists such as neurologists and sleep specialists when possible.

Table 4
Cholinesterase inhibitors: FDA-reported indications, dosage titration, and common adverse effects

Cholinesterase Inhibitors	FDA-Approved Indication	Dosage Titration	Adverse Effects
Donepezil	All stages of AD dementia	*Mild-to-moderate stages (table or orally disintegrating tablet):* 5 mg once daily initially; may increase to 10 mg once daily after 4 to 6 weeks *Moderate-to-severe stage (tablet or orally disintegrating tablet):* 5 mg once daily initially; may increase to 10 mg once daily after 4 to 6 weeks; may increase further to 23 mg once daily if stable on 10 mg once daily for more than 3 months	Nausea, vomiting, diarrhea, loss of appetite, decrease in weight, abnormal dreams, insomnia; caution in patients with bradycardia, respiratory disease, seizure disorder, peptic ulcer disease and urinary tract obstruction
Rivastigmine	Oral: Mild-to-moderate stages of AD dementia Transdermal: all stages of AD dementia	*Capsule:* 1.5 mg twice daily initially; increase by 3 mg daily in every 2 weeks up to 6 mg twice daily *Transdermal patch in mild-to-moderate stages:* 4.6 mg per 24 h initially; increase as tolerated to 9.5 mg per 24 h after 4 weeks; may increase to a maximum dose of 13.3 mg per 24 h after 4 weeks if needed (9.5 mg to 13.3 mg recommended effective dose) *Transdermal patch in severe stage:* Same as in mild-to-moderate stages but target dose is 13.3 mg per 24 h	Nausea, vomiting, diarrhea, loss of appetite, decrease in weight, abnormal dreams, insomnia; caution in patients with bradycardia, respiratory disease, seizure disorder, peptic ulcer disease and urinary tract obstruction Transdermal patch can cause local skin irritation, and reactions (change patch location with each placement to minimize the risk); has less risk of gastrointestinal adverse events compared with oral preparation

(continued on next page)

Table 4
(continued)

Cholinesterase Inhibitors	FDA-Approved Indication	Dosage Titration	Adverse Effects
Galantamine	Mild-to-moderate stages of AD dementia	*Extended-release capsule:* 8 mg once daily for 4 weeks; if tolerated increase to 16 mg once daily for 4 more than 4 weeks; if tolerated increase to 24 mg once daily (recommended target dose range, 16–24 mg once daily) *Immediate-release tablet or solution:* 4 mg twice daily for 4 weeks initially; if tolerated increase to 8 mg twice daily for 4 or more weeks; if tolerated, increase to 12 mg twice daily (recommended target dose range, 16–24 mg daily in two divided doses)	Nausea, vomiting, diarrhea, loss of appetite, decrease in weight, abnormal dreams, insomnia; caution in patients with bradycardia, respiratory disease, seizure disease and peptic ulcer disease and urinary tract obstruction

Table 5
Selected online resource for dementia care

Alzheimer's Association (alz.org)	Offers extensive information, a 24/7 helpline and services for patients with AD and their caregivers. Patient and caregivers can also connect can also connect with local chapters.
National Institute on Aging Information Center (nia.nih.gov/health)	Offers free publications in English and Spanish about aging
Eldercare Locator (eldercare.acl.gov)	A public service of the US administration on Aging that aims to connect patients and caregivers to local support resources such as meals, home care or transportation
NIA Alzheimer's and Related Dementias Education and Referral Center	Offers information on diagnosis, treatment, patient care caregiver needs, long-term care, and research and clinical trials related to AD.

Non-pharmacological treatment

Similar to mNCD/MCI, diet, exercise, and participation in cognitively stimulating leisure activities are also beneficial in the setting of MNCD/dementia.[84,85,103–108] Cognitively stimulating activities should be carefully chosen based on the individual's cognitive abilities as to avoid undue frustration and stress. Reminiscence therapy,[109] music therapy,[110] art therapy,[111] and CST[89] have shown to be of potential benefit to people with dementia by improving quality of life and some even improving cognition.

Owing to the complexity of neurocognitive disorders and its global effect on functionality and health, a collaborative approach with social workers, clinician managers, occupational therapists, nutritionists, speech therapists, physical therapists, palliative care, and others is helpful. Direct collaboration with caregivers is key, and support and education for them should be readily available because of the high caregiver burden of caring for someone with dementia.[112,113] **Table 5** lists online resources for patients and caregivers. Close attention to potential safety issues (ie, driving, proper use of kitchen appliances and furnaces, medication management, access to firearms, elderly abuse), finances, long-term health care planning, medical and advanced care directives, and personal hygiene is essential.[8,114–116] In cases where caregiver support is either not available or insufficient to meet the needs of individuals with dementia, home care, meal services, adult day care programs, respite services, and/or placement in assisted living facilities or skilled nursing facilities should be considered.

A Note on Behavioral and Psychological Symptoms of Dementia

The assessment and treatment of behavioral and psychological symptoms of dementia (BPSD) is paramount. Although pharmacological and non-pharmacological interventions are often deployed, there are no FDA-approved interventions for these symptoms and proper management is often challenging. There are several reviews and meta-analysis focused on the evidence behind these interventions,[117–120] and algorithms for the pharmacological treatment of BPSD.[121,122] Overall, individually tailored non-pharmacological interventions should be trialed first and pharmacological treatments should be tried only when this fails to improve the symptoms.

SUMMARY

Neurocognitive disorders affect dozens of millions of people worldwide carrying a significant burden on society. Although MCI and dementia are characterized by a loss of cognitive abilities, a diagnosis of dementia requires the presence of functional impairment as opposed to patients with MCI who remain independent in their abilities of daily living. The most common type of dementia is due to AD, but other common etiologies include VaD, FTD, DLB, and PDD. In addition to history-taking, cognitive and physical examination, and laboratory workup, neuroimaging, and fluid biomarkers can help with the diagnosis of neurocognitive disorders in clinically challenging cases. Management includes non-pharmacological and pharmacological treatments tailored to the etiology and to the individual. The first-line pharmacological treatment for dementia due to AD is a ChEI with the addition of memantine in the moderate-to-severe stages of the disease. A collaborative approach is key due to the complexity of neurocognitive disorders and its global effect on functionality and health.

DISCLOSURE

No conflicts of interest.

REFERENCES

1. Anderson ND. State of the science on mild cognitive impairment (MCI). CNS Spectr 2019;24(1):78–87.
2. Petersen RC, Lopez O, Armstrong MJ, et al. Practice guideline update summary: mild cognitive impairment: report of the guideline development, dissemination, and implementation subcommittee of the American academy of neurology. Neurology 2018;90(3):126–35.
3. Sanford AM. Mild cognitive impairment. Clin Geriatr Med 2017;33(3):325–37.
4. GBD 2016 Neurology Collaborators. Global, regional, and national burden of neurological disorders, 1990-2016: a systematic analysis for the Global Burden of Disease Study 2016. Lancet Neurol 2019;18(5):459–80.
5. Kramarow EA, Tejada-Vera B. Dementia mortality in the United States, 2000-2017. Natl Vital Stat Rep 2019;68(2):1–29.
6. 2021 Alzheimer's disease facts and figures. Alzheimers Dement J Alzheimers Assoc 2021;17(3):327–406. https://doi.org/10.1002/alz.12328.
7. Akarsu N, Prince MJ, Lawrence V, et al. Depression in carers of people with dementia from a minority ethnic background: Systematic review and meta-analysis of randomised-controlled trials of psychosocial interventions. Int J Geriatr Psychiatry 2019;34(6):790–806.
8. Arvanitakis Z, Shah RC, Bennett DA. Diagnosis and management of dementia: review. JAMA 2019;322(16):1589–99.
9. Livingston G, Huntley J, Sommerlad A, et al. Dementia prevention, intervention, and care: 2020 report of the lancet commission. Lancet Lond Engl 2020; 396(10248):413–46.
10. Hugo J, Ganguli M. Dementia and cognitive impairment: epidemiology, diagnosis, and treatment. Clin Geriatr Med 2014;30(3):421–42.
11. Hogan DB, Fiest KM, Roberts JI, et al. The prevalence and incidence of dementia with Lewy bodies: a systematic review. Can J Neurol Sci J Can Sci Neurol 2016;43(Suppl 1):S83–95.

12. Leroy M, Bertoux M, Skrobala E, et al. Characteristics and progression of patients with frontotemporal dementia in a regional memory clinic network. Alzheimers Res Ther 2021;13(1):19.

13. Young JJ, Lavakumar M, Tampi D, et al. Frontotemporal dementia: latest evidence and clinical implications. Ther Adv Psychopharmacol 2018;8(1):33–48.

14. Vann Jones SA, O'Brien JT. The prevalence and incidence of dementia with Lewy bodies: a systematic review of population and clinical studies. Psychol Med 2014;44(4):673–83.

15. Zaccai J, McCracken C, Brayne C. A systematic review of prevalence and incidence studies of dementia with Lewy bodies. Age Ageing 2005;34(6):561–6.

16. Aarsland D, Zaccai J, Brayne C. A systematic review of prevalence studies of dementia in Parkinson's disease. Mov Disord Off J Mov Disord Soc 2005; 20(10):1255–63.

17. Svenningsson P, Westman E, Ballard C, et al. Cognitive impairment in patients with Parkinson's disease: diagnosis, biomarkers, and treatment. Lancet Neurol 2012;11(8):697–707.

18. Kane JPM, Surendranathan A, Bentley A, et al. Clinical prevalence of Lewy body dementia. Alzheimers Res Ther 2018;10(1):19.

19. Nebel RA, Aggarwal NT, Barnes LL, et al. Understanding the impact of sex and gender in Alzheimer's disease: a call to action. Alzheimers Dement J Alzheimers Assoc 2018;14(9):1171–83.

20. Golub JS, Brickman AM, Ciarleglio AJ, et al. Association of subclinical hearing loss with cognitive performance. JAMA Otolaryngol Head Neck Surg 2020; 146(1):57–67.

21. Avila JF, Rentería MA, Jones RN, et al. Education differentially contributes to cognitive reserve across racial/ethnic groups. Alzheimers Dement 2021;17(1): 70–80.

22. Seraji-Bzorgzad N, Paulson H, Heidebrink J. Neurologic examination in the elderly. Handb Clin Neurol 2019;167:73–88.

23. Elkana O, Tal N, Oren N, et al. Is the cutoff of the MoCA too High? longitudinal data from highly educated older adults. J Geriatr Psychiatry Neurol 2020;33(3): 155–60.

24. Cao L, Hai S, Lin X, et al. Comparison of the saint louis university mental status examination, the mini-mental state examination, and the montreal cognitive assessment in detection of cognitive impairment in chinese elderly from the geriatric department. J Am Med Dir Assoc 2012;13(7):626–9.

25. Cummings-Vaughn LA, Chavakula NN, Malmstrom TK, et al. Veterans affairs saint louis university mental status examination compared with the montreal cognitive assessment and the short test of mental status. J Am Geriatr Soc 2014;62(7):1341–6.

26. Ducharme S, Dols A, Laforce R, et al. Recommendations to distinguish behavioural variant frontotemporal dementia from psychiatric disorders. Brain J Neurol 2020;143(6):1632–50.

27. Silva M de ME, Mercer PBS, Witt MCZ, et al. Olfactory dysfunction in Alzheimer's disease Systematic review and meta-analysis. Dement Neuropsychol 2018; 12(2):123–32.

28. Carnemolla SE, Hsieh JW, Sipione R, et al. Olfactory dysfunction in frontotemporal dementia and psychiatric disorders: a systematic review. Neurosci Biobehav Rev 2020;118:588–611.

29. McKhann GM, Knopman DS, Chertkow H, et al. The diagnosis of dementia due to Alzheimer's disease: recommendations from the National Institute on

Aging-Alzheimer's Association workgroups on diagnostic guidelines for Alzheimer's disease. Alzheimers Dement J Alzheimers Assoc 2011;7(3):263–9.

30. Albert MS, DeKosky ST, Dickson D, et al. The diagnosis of mild cognitive impairment due to Alzheimer's disease: recommendations from the National Institute on Aging-Alzheimer's Association workgroups on diagnostic guidelines for Alzheimer's disease. Alzheimers Dement J Alzheimers Assoc 2011;7(3):270–9.

31. Staffaroni AM, Elahi FM, McDermott D, et al. Neuroimaging in dementia. Semin Neurol 2017;37(5):510–37.

32. Dubois B, Hampel H, Feldman HH, et al. Preclinical Alzheimer's disease: definition, natural history, and diagnostic criteria. Alzheimers Dement J Alzheimers Assoc 2016;12(3):292–323.

33. American Psychiatric Association, editor. Diagnostic and statistical manual of mental disorders: DSM-5. 5th edition. Arlington, VA: American Psychiatric Association; 2013.

34. Gauthier S, Cummings J, Ballard C, et al. Management of behavioral problems in Alzheimer's disease. Int Psychogeriatr 2010;22(3):346–72.

35. Zhao QF, Tan L, Wang HF, et al. The prevalence of neuropsychiatric symptoms in Alzheimer's disease: systematic review and meta-analysis. J Affect Disord 2016; 190:264–71.

36. Jack CR, Bennett DA, Blennow K, et al. NIA-AA research framework: toward a biological definition of Alzheimer's disease. Alzheimers Dement J Alzheimers Assoc 2018;14(4):535–62.

37. Johnson KA, Minoshima S, Bohnen NI, et al. Appropriate use criteria for amyloid PET: a report of the Amyloid Imaging Task Force, the Society of Nuclear Medicine and Molecular Imaging, and the Alzheimer's Association. Alzheimers Dement J Alzheimers Assoc 2013;9(1):e-1–16.

38. Masters CL, Bateman R, Blennow K, et al. Alzheimer's disease. Nat Rev Dis Primer 2015;1:15056.

39. Zhu XC, Tan L, Wang HF, et al. Rate of early onset Alzheimer's disease: a systematic review and meta-analysis. Ann Transl Med 2015;3(3):38.

40. Goldman JS, Hahn SE, Catania JW, et al. Genetic counseling and testing for Alzheimer disease: joint practice guidelines of the American College of Medical Genetics and the National Society of Genetic Counselors. Genet Med 2011; 13(6):597–605.

41. Rentería ME, Mitchell BL, de Lara AM. Genetic testing for Alzheimer's disease: trends, challenges and ethical considerations. Curr Opin Psychiatry 2020;33(2): 136–40.

42. Jellinger KA, Attems J. Is there pure vascular dementia in old age? J Neurol Sci 2010;299(1–2):150–4.

43. Reed BR, Mungas DM, Kramer JH, et al. Profiles of neuropsychological impairment in autopsy-defined Alzheimer's disease and cerebrovascular disease. Brain J Neurol 2007;130(Pt 3):731–9.

44. Graff-Radford J. Vascular cognitive impairment. Contin Minneap Minn 2019; 25(1):147–64.

45. Baezner H, Blahak C, Poggesi A, et al. Association of gait and balance disorders with age-related white matter changes: the LADIS study. Neurology 2008;70(12):935–42.

46. Schmidt R, Berghold A, Jokinen H, et al. White matter lesion progression in LADIS: frequency, clinical effects, and sample size calculations. Stroke 2012; 43(10):2643–7.

47. Salmon DP, Filoteo JV. Neuropsychology of cortical versus subcortical dementia syndromes. Semin Neurol 2007;27(1):7–21.
48. Charidimou A, Peeters A, Fox Z, et al. Spectrum of transient focal neurological episodes in cerebral amyloid angiopathy: multicentre magnetic resonance imaging cohort study and meta-analysis. Stroke 2012;43(9):2324–30.
49. Arvanitakis Z, Leurgans SE, Wang Z, et al. Cerebral amyloid angiopathy pathology and cognitive domains in older persons. Ann Neurol 2011;69(2):320–7.
50. Peters N, Opherk C, Danek A, et al. The pattern of cognitive performance in CADASIL: a Monogenic condition leading to subcortical ischemic vascular dementia. Am J Psychiatry 2005;162(11):2078–85.
51. Hara K, Shiga A, Fukutake T, et al. Association of HTRA1 mutations and familial ischemic cerebral small-vessel disease. N Engl J Med 2009;360(17):1729–39.
52. Revesz T, Holton JL, Lashley T, et al. Genetics and molecular pathogenesis of sporadic and hereditary cerebral amyloid angiopathies. Acta Neuropathol (Berl) 2009;118(1):115–30.
53. Tomidokoro Y, Rostagno A, Neubert TA, et al. Iowa variant of familial Alzheimer's disease: accumulation of posttranslationally modified AbetaD23N in parenchymal and cerebrovascular amyloid deposits. Am J Pathol 2010;176(4): 1841–54.
54. Zhang-Nunes SX, Maat-Schieman MLC, van Duinen SG, et al. The cerebral beta-amyloid angiopathies: hereditary and sporadic. Brain Pathol Zurich Switz 2006;16(1):30–9.
55. Rascovsky K, Hodges JR, Knopman D, et al. Sensitivity of revised diagnostic criteria for the behavioural variant of frontotemporal dementia. Brain J Neurol 2011;134(Pt 9):2456–77.
56. Diehl-Schmid J, Grimmer T, Drzezga A, et al. Decline of cerebral glucose metabolism in frontotemporal dementia: a longitudinal 18F-FDG-PET-study. Neurobiol Aging 2007;28(1):42–50.
57. Padovani A, Agosti C, Premi E, et al. Extrapyramidal symptoms in Frontotemporal Dementia: prevalence and clinical correlations. Neurosci Lett 2007;422(1): 39–42.
58. Park HK, Park KH, Yoon B, et al. Clinical characteristics of parkinsonism in frontotemporal dementia according to subtypes. J Neurol Sci 2017;372:51–6.
59. Gorno-Tempini ML, Hillis AE, Weintraub S, et al. Classification of primary progressive aphasia and its variants. Neurology 2011;76(11):1006–14.
60. Montembeault M, Brambati SM, Gorno-Tempini ML, et al. Clinical, anatomical, and pathological features in the three variants of primary progressive aphasia: a review. Front Neurol 2018;9:692.
61. Giannini LAA, Irwin DJ, McMillan CT, et al. Clinical marker for Alzheimer disease pathology in logopenic primary progressive aphasia. Neurology 2017;88(24): 2276–84.
62. Ossenkoppele R, Schonhaut DR, Schöll M, et al. Tau PET patterns mirror clinical and neuroanatomical variability in Alzheimer's disease. Brain 2016;139(5): 1551–67.
63. Villarejo-Galende A, Llamas-Velasco S, Gómez-Grande A, et al. Amyloid pet in primary progressive aphasia: case series and systematic review of the literature. J Neurol 2017;264(1):121–30.
64. Rohrer JD, Guerreiro R, Vandrovcova J, et al. The heritability and genetics of frontotemporal lobar degeneration. Neurology 2009;73(18):1451–6.
65. Chow TW, Miller BL, Hayashi VN, et al. Inheritance of frontotemporal dementia. Arch Neurol 1999;56(7):817–22.

66. Goldman JS, Farmer JM, Wood EM, et al. Comparison of family histories in FTLD subtypes and related tauopathies. Neurology 2005;65(11):1817–9.

67. Seelaar H, Kamphorst W, Rosso SM, et al. Distinct genetic forms of frontotemporal dementia. Neurology 2008;71(16):1220–6.

68. Sezgin M, Bilgic B, Tinaz S, et al. Parkinson's disease dementia and Lewy body disease. Semin Neurol 2019;39(2):274–82.

69. McKeith IG, Boeve BF, Dickson DW, et al. Diagnosis and management of dementia with Lewy bodies: Fourth consensus report of the DLB Consortium. Neurology 2017;89(1):88–100.

70. Hamilton JM, Landy KM, Salmon DP, et al. Early visuospatial deficits predict the occurrence of visual hallucinations in autopsy-confirmed dementia with Lewy Bodies. Am J Geriatr Psychiatry 2012;20(9):773–81.

71. Postuma RB, Gagnon JF, Vendette M, et al. Quantifying the risk of neurodegenerative disease in idiopathic REM sleep behavior disorder. Neurology 2009; 72(15):1296–300.

72. Day GS, Scarmeas N, Dubinsky R, et al. Aducanumab use in symptomatic Alzheimer disease evidence in focus: a report of the AAN guidelines subcommittee. Neurology 2022;98(15):619–31.

73. Cooper C, Li R, Lyketsos C, et al. Treatment for mild cognitive impairment: systematic review. Br J Psychiatry J Ment Sci 2013;203(3):255–64.

74. Petersen RC, Thomas RG, Grundman M, et al. Vitamin E and donepezil for the treatment of mild cognitive impairment. N Engl J Med 2005;352(23):2379–88.

75. Raschetti R, Albanese E, Vanacore N, et al. Cholinesterase inhibitors in mild cognitive impairment: a systematic review of randomised trials. PLoS Med 2007;4(11):e338.

76. Cheng D, Kong H, Pang W, et al. B vitamin supplementation improves cognitive function in the middle aged and elderly with hyperhomocysteinemia. Nutr Neurosci 2016;19(10):461–6.

77. Li MM, Yu JT, Wang HF, et al. Efficacy of vitamins B supplementation on mild cognitive impairment and Alzheimer's disease: a systematic review and meta-analysis. Curr Alzheimer Res 2014;11(9):844–52.

78. Krause D, Roupas P. Effect of vitamin intake on cognitive decline in older adults: evaluation of the evidence. J Nutr Health Aging 2015;19(7):745–53.

79. Snitz BE, O'Meara ES, Carlson MC, et al. Ginkgo biloba for preventing cognitive decline in older adults: a randomized trial. JAMA 2009;302(24):2663–70.

80. Naeini AMA, Elmadfa I, Djazayery A, et al. The effect of antioxidant vitamins E and C on cognitive performance of the elderly with mild cognitive impairment in Isfahan, Iran: a double-blind, randomized, placebo-controlled trial. Eur J Nutr 2014;53(5):1255–62.

81. Singh B, Parsaik AK, Mielke MM, et al. Association of mediterranean diet with mild cognitive impairment and Alzheimer's disease: a systematic review and meta-analysis. J Alzheimers Dis JAD 2014;39(2):271–82.

82. Morris MC, Tangney CC, Wang Y, et al. MIND diet associated with reduced incidence of Alzheimer's disease. Alzheimers Dement J Alzheimers Assoc 2015; 11(9):1007–14.

83. Kheirouri S, Alizadeh M. MIND diet and cognitive performance in older adults: a systematic review. Crit Rev Food Sci Nutr 2021;1–19. https://doi.org/10.1080/10408398.2021.1925220.

84. Hosking DE, Eramudugolla R, Cherbuin N, et al. MIND not Mediterranean diet related to 12-year incidence of cognitive impairment in an Australian longitudinal cohort study. Alzheimers Dement J Alzheimers Assoc 2019;15(4):581–9.

85. Nuzum H, Stickel A, Corona M, et al. Potential benefits of physical activity in MCI and dementia. Behav Neurol 2020;2020:7807856.
86. Butler M, McCreedy E, Nelson VA, et al. Does cognitive training prevent cognitive decline?: A systematic review. Ann Intern Med 2018;168(1):63–8.
87. Hall CB, Lipton RB, Sliwinski M, et al. Cognitive activities delay onset of memory decline in persons who develop dementia. Neurology 2009;73(5):356–61.
88. Altschul DM, Deary IJ. Playing analog games is associated with reduced declines in cognitive function: a 68-year longitudinal cohort study. J Gerontol Ser B 2020;75(3):474–82.
89. Rai H, Yates L, Orrell M. Cognitive stimulation therapy for dementia. Clin Geriatr Med 2018;34(4):653–65.
90. Gomez-Soria I, Peralta-Marrupe P, Plo F. Cognitive stimulation program in mild cognitive impairment a randomized controlled trial. Dement Neuropsychol 2020;14(2):110–7.
91. Cummings JL, Tong G, Ballard C. Treatment combinations for Alzheimer's disease: current and future pharmacotherapy options. J Alzheimers Dis JAD 2019;67(3):779–94.
92. Birks J, Harvey RJ. Donepezil for dementia due to Alzheimer's disease. Cochrane Database Syst Rev 2006;1:CD001190.
93. Schmidt R, Hofer E, Bouwman FH, et al. EFNS-ENS/EAN Guideline on concomitant use of cholinesterase inhibitors and memantine in moderate to severe Alzheimer's disease. Eur J Neurol 2015;22(6):889–98.
94. Matsunaga S, Kishi T, Iwata N. Combination therapy with cholinesterase inhibitors and memantine for Alzheimer's disease: a systematic review and meta-analysis. Int J Neuropsychopharmacol 2015;18(5):pyu115.
95. Battle CE, Abdul-Rahim AH, Shenkin SD, et al. Cholinesterase inhibitors for vascular dementia and other vascular cognitive impairments: a network meta-analysis. Cochrane Database Syst Rev 2021;2:CD013306.
96. McShane R, Westby MJ, Roberts E, et al. Memantine for dementia. Cochrane Database Syst Rev 2019;3. https://doi.org/10.1002/14651858.CD003154.pub6.
97. O'Brien JT, Thomas A. Vascular dementia. Lancet 2015;386(10004):1698–706.
98. Sivasathiaseelan H, Marshall CR, Agustus JL, et al. Frontotemporal dementia: a clinical review. Semin Neurol 2019;39(2):251–63.
99. Mendez MF, Shapira JS, McMurtray A, et al. Preliminary findings: behavioral worsening on donepezil in patients with frontotemporal dementia. Am J Geriatr Psychiatry 2007;15(1):84–7. https://doi.org/10.1097/01.JGP.0000231744.69631.33.
100. Stinton C, McKeith I, Taylor JP, et al. Pharmacological management of Lewy body dementia: a systematic review and meta-analysis. Am J Psychiatry 2015;172(8):731–42.
101. Wang HF, Yu JT, Tang SW, et al. Efficacy and safety of cholinesterase inhibitors and memantine in cognitive impairment in Parkinson's disease, Parkinson's disease dementia, and dementia with Lewy bodies: systematic review with meta-analysis and trial sequential analysis. J Neurol Neurosurg Psychiatr 2015;86(2):135–43.
102. Taylor JP, McKeith IG, Burn DJ, et al. New evidence on the management of Lewy body dementia. Lancet Neurol 2020;19(2):157–69.
103. Cheng ST, Chow PK, Song YQ, et al. Mental and physical activities delay cognitive decline in older persons with dementia. Am J Geriatr Psychiatry 2014;22(1):63–74.

104. Rebok GW, Ball K, Guey LT, et al. Ten-year effects of the advanced cognitive training for independent and vital elderly cognitive training trial on cognition and everyday functioning in older adults. J Am Geriatr Soc 2014;62(1):16–24.
105. Hoffmann K, Sobol NA, Frederiksen KS, et al. Moderate-to-high intensity physical exercise in patients with Alzheimer's disease: a randomized controlled trial. J Alzheimers Dis JAD 2016;50(2):443–53.
106. Pitkälä KH, Pöysti MM, Laakkonen ML, et al. Effects of the finnish alzheimer disease exercise trial (FINALEX): a randomized controlled trial. JAMA Intern Med 2013;173(10):894–901.
107. Sink KM, Espeland MA, Castro CM, et al. Effect of a 24-month physical activity intervention vs health education on cognitive outcomes in sedentary older adults: the LIFE randomized trial. JAMA 2015;314(8):781–90.
108. Lamb SE, Sheehan B, Atherton N, et al. Dementia And Physical Activity (DAPA) trial of moderate to high intensity exercise training for people with dementia: randomised controlled trial. BMJ 2018;361:k1675.
109. Wang JJ. Group reminiscence therapy for cognitive and affective function of demented elderly in Taiwan. Int J Geriatr Psychiatry 2007;22(12):1235–40.
110. Lam HL, Li WTV, Laher I, et al. Effects of music therapy on patients with dementia-a systematic review. Geriatr Basel Switz 2020;5(4):E62.
111. Emblad SYM, Mukaetova-Ladinska EB. Creative art therapy as a non-pharmacological intervention for dementia: a systematic review. J Alzheimers Dis Rep 2021;5(1):353–64.
112. Connors MH, Seeher K, Teixeira-Pinto A, et al. Dementia and caregiver burden: a three-year longitudinal study. Int J Geriatr Psychiatry 2020;35(2):250–8.
113. Adelman RD, Tmanova LL, Delgado D, et al. Caregiver burden: a clinical review. JAMA 2014;311(10):1052–60.
114. Thyrian JR, Hertel J, Wucherer D, et al. Effectiveness and safety of dementia care management in primary care: a randomized clinical trial. JAMA Psychiatry 2017;74(10):996–1004.
115. Laakkonen ML, Kautiainen H, Hölttä E, et al. Effects of self-management groups for people with dementia and their spouses–randomized controlled trial. J Am Geriatr Soc 2016;64(4):752–60.
116. Widera E, Steenpass V, Marson D, et al. Finances in the older patient with cognitive impairment: "He didn't want me to take over. JAMA 2011;305(7):698–706.
117. Abraha I, Rimland JM, Trotta FM, et al. Systematic review of systematic reviews of non-pharmacological interventions to treat behavioural disturbances in older patients with dementia. The SENATOR-OnTop series. BMJ Open 2017;7(3): e012759.
118. Bessey LJ, Walaszek A. Management of behavioral and psychological symptoms of dementia. Curr Psychiatry Rep 2019;21(8):66.
119. Yunusa I, Alsumali A, Garba AE, et al. Assessment of reported comparative effectiveness and safety of atypical antipsychotics in the treatment of behavioral and psychological symptoms of dementia: a network meta-analysis. JAMA Netw Open 2019;2(3):e190828.
120. Tampi RR, Tampi DJ, Rogers K, et al. Antipsychotics in the management of behavioral and psychological symptoms of dementia: maximizing gain and minimizing harm. Neurodegener Dis Manag 2020;10(1):5–8.
121. Chen A, Copeli F, Metzger E, et al. The psychopharmacology algorithm project at the harvard south shore program: an update on management of behavioral and psychological symptoms in dementia. Psychiatry Res 2021;295:113641.

122. Davies SJ, Burhan AM, Kim D, et al. Sequential drug treatment algorithm for agitation and aggression in Alzheimer's and mixed dementia. J Psychopharmacol Oxf Engl 2018;32(5):509–23.
123. McCollum L, Karlawish J. Cognitive Impairment Evaluation and Management. Med Clin North Am 2020;104(5):807–25.
124. Morris JC. Clinical dementia rating: a reliable and valid diagnostic and staging measure for dementia of the Alzheimer type 1997;9(1):173–8.

Pathophysiology of Alzheimer's Disease

Brandon C. Yarns, MD, MS[a,b,]*, Kelsey A. Holiday, PhD[a], David M. Carlson, MD[a,b], Coleman K. Cosgrove, DO, PhD[c,1], Rebecca J. Melrose, PhD[a,b]

KEYWORDS

- Alzheimer's disease • Dementia • Pathophysiology • Amyloid • Tau • Aducanumb

KEY POINTS

- Alzheimer's disease (AD) is the most common cause of dementia worldwide.
- Aggregates of amyloid and tau proteins are the pathophysiologic hallmark of AD but its exact mechanisms remain a topic of ongoing investigation.
- Numerous risk and protective factors interact with pathophysiologic mechanisms and cultural factors, such as race and ethnicity in AD.
- Biomarker and neuroimaging research has demonstrated how AD pathologic processes may lead to cognitive and neuropsychiatric symptoms.
- As the pathophysiology behind AD gains clarity, more potential treatment options are emerging.

INTRODUCTION

Alzheimer's disease (AD) is a neurodegenerative process often leading to dementia, affecting 12% of women and 9% of men over age 65.[1] People with dementia have profound cognitive deficits that represent a decline from premorbid levels of functioning and interfere with their ability to complete important self-care activities.[2] While there is variability, most patients with AD initially present with deficits in memory that extend to include deficits in language, visuospatial functioning, and executive functioning. In addition, neuropsychiatric symptoms emerge in 97% of patients, particularly in later stages.[3] Numerous neuropathological processes disrupt the functioning and integrity of neurons. A common model of AD posits that neuropathological processes lead to

[a] Psychiatry/Mental Health Service, VA Greater Los Angeles Healthcare System, 11301 Wilshire Boulevard, Building 401, Mail Code 116AE, Los Angeles, CA 90073, USA; [b] Department of Psychiatry and Biobehavioral Sciences, David Geffen School of Medicine at UCLA, 757 Westwood Plaza #4, Los Angeles, CA 90095, USA; [c] Department of Psychiatry, University at Buffalo, 462 Grider Street, Buffalo, NY 14215, USA
[1] Present address: 462 Grider Street, Buffalo, NY 14215.
* Corresponding author. 11301 Wilshire Boulevard, Building 401, Mail Code 116AE, Los Angeles, CA 90073.
E-mail address: BYarns@mednet.ucla.edu

Psychiatr Clin N Am 45 (2022) 663–676
https://doi.org/10.1016/j.psc.2022.07.003
0193-953X/22/Published by Elsevier Inc.

neuronal cell loss, leading to cognitive deficits and a loss of functional independence. In this review, we discuss the neuropathological process of AD, risk and protective factors, the association between pathology/neuronal damage and the clinical symptoms of AD, and treatment implications.

PATHOPHYSIOLOGIC MECHANISMS

The neuropathologic hallmarks of AD are plaques formed around deposits of extracellular amyloid beta (Aβ) proteins and neurofibrillary tangles (NFT) of accumulated hyperphosphorylated tau protein. However, recent analyses have identified numerous hypothesized processes contributing to the onset of AD.[4] Though there have been efforts toward a unifying hypothesis,[5] the pathogenesis of AD remains a topic of extensive investigation.

Amyloid Hypothesis

Amyloid plaques (also called neuritic or senile plaques) are formed by abnormal proteolytic cleavage of amyloid precursor protein (APP), a membrane protein produced in the endoplasmic reticulum and transported to the Golgi complex for cleavage by any of three secretases: α, β, or γ. Cleavage by α secretase produces amyloid with a soluble extracellular domain that may be neuroprotective.[6] Cleavage by β or γ secretase gives rise to Aβ fragments ranging in size from 39 to 43 amino acids, most commonly $A\beta_{1-40}$ and $A\beta_{1-42}$. Further, $A\beta_{1-40}$ is soluble, less neurotoxic, and found in healthy brains, whereas $A\beta_{1-42}$ has a hydrophobic extracellular domain that interacts with numerous extracellular components to form plaques. There have been reports over the past decade of an $A\beta_{1-43}$ cleavage product that is highly neurotoxic and more amyloidogenic than the shorter products.[7] These amyloid plaques lead to interactions that contribute to further neuronal loss and the progression of AD.[5]

Tau/Neurofibrillary Tangles Hypothesis

Tau is a microtubule protein in neuronal cells that stabilizes the microtubular assembly and thus plays a central role in neuronal development and axonal growth. Normally, a balance of phosphorylated and dephosphorylated tau is maintained by a group of tau phosphatases and microtubule-associated kinases.[8] However, in pathologic conditions, upregulation of kinases and downregulation of phosphatases cause hyperphosphorylation of tau that results in insoluble double-helical filaments, leading to the formation of protein complexes/clumps known as NFT. These NFTs lead to the degeneration of neurons and synaptic dysfunction, and they survive even after the death of the affected neurons, when they are released extracellularly and interact with astrocytes and microglia. In AD, NFTs are predominantly found within the hippocampus, the entorhinal cortex, amygdala, dorsal raphae, and nucleus basalis of Meynert.[9,10]

Cerebrovascular Disease

Vascular factors and cognitive impairment are repeatedly linked in dementia, including AD.[11] As diagnostic criteria for AD and vascular dementia are somewhat loosely defined, a mixed type of vascular and AD is frequently encountered.[12] Reduced cerebral blood flow may drive this connection between cerebrovascular disease (CVD) and AD risk.[13] Arterial stiffness may also mediate the link between CVD and dementia, as it correlates with Aβ deposition and disease progression.[14–16] A synergistic relationship exists between CVD risk factors, Aβ, and tau in people with AD, such that CVD may increase Aβ and tau accumulation, which in turn induces microvascular damage in the brain.[17–19]

Neurotransmitters

Cholinergic System

While multiple neurotransmitter systems are affected in AD, the cholinergic system was the earliest hypothesized contributor and the target of most available pharmacotherapies.[20] There are two classes of acetylcholine receptors in the brain: muscarinic receptors, predominantly found in the hippocampus, cortex, and thalamus; and nicotinic receptors, mostly in the striatum, cortex, superior colliculus, cerebellum, and thalamus.[21] There is extensive evidence that disruption of both types of cholinergic transmission contributes to the pathology and deficits seen in AD.[22] In particular, nicotinic receptor binding is reduced in specific limbic and subcortical regions in mild cognitive impairment (MCI) and further reduced in AD dementia compared to cognitively unimpaired adults and is related to cognitive deficits and neuropsychiatric symptoms.[23,24]

Serotonergic System

Degeneration of serotonergic neurons and hypofunction of the serotonergic (5-hydroxytryptamine) system, particularly in the hippocampus, has been shown to play a role in behavioral aspects of AD.[25,26] Based on animal models, 5-HT6 and 5-HT7 receptors may have a role in the learning and memory deficits seen in AD.[27,28]

Glutamatergic System

Excitotoxicity of glutamatergic receptors, particularly N-Methyl-D-aspartate (NMDA), is thought to play a key role in AD development due to glutamate's action as a physiologic substrate for memory function and its contribution to the production of amyloid plaques and neuronal loss.[29,30] NMDA antagonism is the mechanism of action of memantine, one of the few the Food and Drug Administration (FDA)-approved drug therapies for AD.[31]

Dopaminergic System

Though dopamine is less sensitive to Aβ toxicity than acetylcholine or serotonin, dopamine's association with learning, memory, and motivation suggests a potential role for dopaminergic signaling in AD.[32,33] Deficiencies in dopamine may underpin apathy in AD.[34] Downregulation of dopaminergic receptors could also explain the presence of extrapyramidal symptoms in AD.[35]

Other Possible Mechanisms

Inflammation

Both amyloid plaques and NFT interact with and can activate microglia and astrocytes, leading to a neuroinflammatory cascade.[36] As astrocytes bind to Aβ sites, they secrete proinflammatory mediators, including interleukins, prostaglandins, leukotrienes, and thromboxanes. Activation of microglia leads to increased expression of proinflammatory cytokines, including interleukin-1β, interleukin-6, TNF-α, and interleukin-8.[6,37]

Oxidative stress

Aβ plaques interfere with the electron transport chain, producing multiple reactive oxygen species that can damage cellular components and interfere with DNA at a structural level.[38]

Epigenetics

Evidence suggests that epigenetic modifications lead to altered gene expression at a transcriptional level in AD.[6] Examples include DNA methylation and hydroxymethylation, noncoding RNA regulation, histone post-translational modifications, and lower mitochondrial DNA copy number associated with AD pathophysiology.[39]

PATHOPHYSIOLOGY AND RISK AND PROTECTIVE FACTORS

Numerous risk and protective factors are associated with AD, but these should be understood to vary across cultural groups, defined as ethnicity, race, native languages, and country of origin.[40] Cultural differences in values, knowledge, and conventions of communication influence performance on cognitive assessments.[41] According to research, Hispanic Americans with AD have an earlier onset than other groups,[42] which may be due to lower socioeconomic status, education level/quality, English language proficiency, country of origin, level of acculturation, and perceived discrimination.[42,43] When compared with non-Hispanic whites, black Americans evidenced a twofold greater prevalence and incidence of AD, a slower rate of cognitive decline, and a higher prevalence of genetic risk factors (eg, APOE4 allele).[44–46] In addition to differences between racial and ethnic groups, there is heterogeneity in disease incidence, onset, and progression in subpopulations *within* these groups.[40] Yet, racial/ethnic communities that are disproportionately affected by AD (eg, blacks, Latinx) are routinely underrepresented in research studies and clinical trials.[42,47,48] Our understanding of risk and the protective factors that follow should be viewed through this lens.

Age

Age has been consistently identified as one of the most important demographic risk factors for cognitive impairment and AD,[49,50] and the prevalence of AD doubles every 5 years past the age of 65.[51] The mechanisms of brain aging suggested to increase the risk of AD include mitochondrial dysfunction, glucose hypometabolism, immune/inflammatory reactions, Aβ, dyslipidemia, white matter degeneration, and decreased regeneration.[52]

Genetics

The apolipoprotein E-e4 (APOE4) allele on chromosome 19 has been consistently identified as a risk factor for AD, and over 60% of people with AD carry this allele.[52,53] APOE4, a cholesterol transporter important for myelin and neuronal membrane maintenance in the brain,[54] has been linked to increased Aβ[55] and impaired Aβ clearance.[56] In contrast to late or "typical" onset AD, early onset AD (age <65 years) is rare and has been strongly associated with familial mutations in APP and presenilin genes.[49]

Sex

Women have an increased risk of AD compared with men; 60% of people with AD are female.[52,57] There seems to be a complex interplay between sex, age, and genetics in AD. Carrying the APOE4 allele confers an increased risk of acquiring AD for women compared with men, particularly for women who are heterozygous, carrying only one APOE4 allele.[52,53] In contrast, men who are *homo*zygous for the APOE4 allele have an increased risk of developing cognitive impairment after acquiring AD compared with homozygous women.[52,58]

Traumatic Brain Injury

A history of traumatic brain injury (TBI) has been identified as a risk factor for AD.[59–62] Some studies link TBI to AD pathology, such as NFT.[63,64] Other studies suggest that TBIs have a synergistic effect on pre-existing genetic risk factors for AD (eg, APOE4 alleles)[65] or upregulate APP.[59] Additionally, TBIs may induce cerebrovascular pathology[66] or metabolic dysfunction.[67] The impact of TBI on AD may differ across populations; one study found that a history of TBI with loss of consciousness was associated with a 2–3-year earlier-onset AD dementia for white and black Americans and a 6-year earlier onset in Hispanic males.[68] In contrast, other studies have not found a significant relationship between TBI and the clinical presentation of AD or AD pathology.[69–72]

Lifestyle and Environmental Factors

In addition to a possible pathophysiologic mechanism, CVD is one of the major acquired risk factors for AD.[73,74] There are strong associations between CVD risk and lifestyle factors that are shaped by cultural and lifespan experiences. A study on the global epidemiology of dementia found that low educational attainment and other socioeconomic factors were associated with elevated CVD risk factors including obesity, sedentarism, diabetes, hypertension, dyslipidemia, and metabolic syndrome and subsequently an increased risk of developing AD.[75]

Smoking, sleep disturbance, and chronic stress are risk factors for AD.[73] Cigarette smoking has been associated with cerebral oxidative stress and an increased risk and earlier onset of AD.[76] Sleep disturbances have been found to increase systemic inflammation and, subsequently, Aβ burden.[77] Chronic stress has been associated with increased CVD and elevated glucocorticoid levels.[78,79] A systematic review of over 60 environmental risk factors for dementia found moderate evidence for air pollution (eg, particulates, ozone), aluminum, silicon, pesticides, and electromagnetic fields as risk factors for AD dementia.[74]

Protective Factors

The Lancet Commission revealed that one in three dementia cases could be prevented by modifying lifestyle risk factors, including hypertension, diabetes, obesity, and physical activity.[80] Increased physical activity has been associated with a decreased risk of CVD, AD, and AD pathology.[81] Furthermore, adherence to a Mediterranean diet (ie, high intake of fruits, vegetables, fish, and olive oil) has been associated with a decreased risk of developing AD and of MCI progressing to AD.[82]

Cognitive Reserve

Higher levels of education have been associated with a reduced risk of AD[83] and slower cognitive decline.[84] The Cognitive Reserve model suggests that high levels of education produce a "cognitive reserve" that can compensate for AD pathology via processes, such as more efficient utilization of brain networks or recruiting alternative brain networks.[85,86] In addition, people with high levels of "brain reserve" have larger brain volumes that can reduce the presentation of clinical symptoms associated with damage to these regions.[87,88] The impact of cognitive reserve, however, may not be universal across racial and ethnic groups. One study found that higher levels of education buffered the impact of white matter burden and cortical thinning in white but not black or Hispanic individuals.[89] Relatedly, bilingualism has been associated with a delayed onset of dementia and better cognitive performance than predicted by brain structure or level of pathology.[90]

PATHOPHYSIOLOGY AND SYMPTOMS

Our understanding of how AD pathologic processes may lead to cognitive and neuropsychiatric symptoms comes primarily from biomarker or neuroimaging research. In classic AD, mesial temporal lobe (MTL) atrophy is observed on structural imaging, such as MRI or highly sensitive computerized tomography scans.[91] Brain functioning can be assessed using fluorodeoxyglucose-PET. AD is characterized by decreased glucose metabolism in superior and posterior temporal regions, parietal lobes, posterior cingulate cortex, and the precuneus.[91]

Cognitive Deficits

The most common presentation of cognitive deficits in AD is the amnestic presentation,[92] which is defined as impaired encoding or consolidation of information such that retrieval cues do not facilitate memory performance.[93] Memories in people with AD tend to have a temporal gradient with greater impairments for recent than for remote memories.[94,95] Amnestic deficits are associated with MTL atrophy, including in the hippocampus and entorhinal cortex,[91,96] loss of cholinergic receptor binding in the hippocampus,[23] and accumulation of tau in MTL.[97]

In addition to the pronounced episodic memory declines in amnestic AD, deficits in executive functioning are commonly detected early in the disease process.[96] Executive function deficits include difficulties with planning, multitasking, sustained attention, inhibition, problem-solving, and cognitive flexibility.[98] Executive dysfunction in AD has been linked to damage to the prefrontal cortex,[99] and parietal and temporal cortex.[100] Higher NFT counts in the hippocampus, inferior parietal cortex, and superior temporal cortex were associated with poorer performance on a measure of inhibition,[101] whereas an association with amyloid is indeterminate.[102] The heterogeneity of executive dysfunction and corresponding neuroanatomical correlates in AD may be due to the large cortical network associated with executive functioning and patterns that vary by disease severity.[103]

Impairments in language, especially object naming in AD, have been associated with abnormalities in temporal,[104] frontal, and parietal cortex.[105,106] Verbal fluency, or the ability to generate words based on a rule,[107] is also impacted. Patients with AD have greater deficits in semantic fluency (eg, naming animals) than in phonemic fluency (eg, naming words beginning with a specific letter),[95,107] and this greater deficit in semantic fluency is associated with temporal regions' degradation. [107]

The most common visuospatial problems in AD include deficits in spatial orientation (eg, reaching for objects), visual localization (eg, finding objects in space), navigation, reading, and hand–eye coordination.[108] Aβ, tau, and neuroinflammation may induce changes in the visual system in cortical (particularly temporal and parietal regions) and subcortical regions, peripheral nerves, and even structures in the eye.[109]

Neuropsychiatric Symptoms

Neuropsychiatric symptoms affect up to 97% of individuals with dementia and impair quality of life and activities of daily living, leading to earlier institutionalization, faster disease progression, increased mortality, and caregiver stress.[3]

Depression is among the most frequent neuropsychiatric complications of AD and affects up to 50% of patients.[110] Aβ plaques and NFT are more pronounced in the brains of AD patients with comorbid depression compared with those without depression.[111] Chronic inflammation, hypothalamic–pituitary–adrenal (HPA) axis hyperactivation, and neurotrophin signaling deficits appear to be common pathophysiological mechanisms between AD and depression.[111] Apathy, a similar yet distinct symptom, is associated with faster cognitive and functional decline, suggesting that apathy in AD is associated with a more aggressive dementia.[112] Apathy and anxiety are related to Aβ deposition.[113] Apathy is also associated with increased anterior cingulate NFT burden[114] and bilateral anterior cingulate and left medial frontal cortex atrophy.[115]

Psychotic symptoms (delusions and hallucinations) in AD have prevalence rates ranging from 10% to 73%, with a median of 34% within the clinic setting and 7% to 20% in the community and clinical trials.[116] A robust body of research has indicated that AD with psychosis is associated with impaired frontal lobe function.[117]

Aggression may be linked with serotonergic dysfunction.[118] Agitation is associated with NFT burden in the orbitofrontal and anterior cingulate cortices.[119]

PATHOPHSYIOLOGY AND TREATMENT

Current pharmacologic treatment options for cognition and global functioning in AD target the cholinergic and glutamatergic systems. Acetylcholinesterase inhibitors—donepezil, galantamine, rivastigmine, and tacrine—target the acetylcholine deficit arising from hypofunction in the nucleus basalis of Meynert by inhibiting the enzyme that degrades acetylcholine within the synapse.[120] Memantine is the sole NMDA receptor antagonist approved for use in AD and should be reserved for moderate-severe symptoms.[31] These drugs have a modest but clinically significant benefit for symptomatic management but do not alter the clinical trajectory.

In June 2021, the FDA approved aducanumab, the first novel medication to treat AD in over 25 years.[121] Aducanumab is a human immunoglobulin gamma 1 monoclonal antibody directed against aggregated Aβ approved for the treatment of mild AD. While its approval is based on reduction of Aβ in the brain—a potential disease-modifying treatment strategy—controversy remains because of the failure to meet clinical endpoints in all aducanumab trials, concerns about cost-effectiveness, potential adverse effects, including amyloid-related imaging abnormalities, and critiques of the amyloid hypothesis.

As the pathophysiology behind the disease gains clarity, more potential treatment options are emerging. Several emerging options target Aβ plaques, including APP-cleaving enzyme inhibitors (beta-site amyloid precursor protein (APP)-cleaving enzyme [BACE] inhibitors), Aβ monoclonal antibodies, and Aβ vaccines.[122] Treatments that target tau aggregates include active and passive immunizations, inhibitors of tyrosine kinase, receptor for advanced glycation end-products inhibitors, and tyrosine kinase inhibitors.[122] Evidence supports possible combination therapy using these modalities, though further research is needed.[123,124]

SUMMARY

The pathophysiology of AD is primarily centered on the development and propagation of Aβ proteins and NFT that lead to neuronal dysfunction and, ultimately, the clinical symptoms of dementia. Research continues exploring the additive or interactive impact of CVD, inflammation, oxidative stress, and epigenetics on disease progression. Although approximately 70% of the risk of AD is attributable to genetics,[73] a wide range of cultural, lifestyle, and environmental factors influence its pathophysiology. The development of cognitive and neuropsychiatric symptoms of AD is closely correlated with pathophysiologic brain changes. As research expands the knowledge of AD pathophysiology, more treatments are anticipated to emerge that modify the disease process to relieve the burden of AD worldwide.

CLINICS CARE POINTS

- Alzheimer's disease (AD) is a neurodegenerative process often leading to dementia that affects 12% of women and 9% of men over age 65.
- Neuritic plaques of extracellular amyloid beta (Aβ) proteins and neurofibrillary tangles of accumulated hyperphosphorylated tau protein are the pathophysiologic hallmarks of AD. However, its exact pathogenesis remains a topic of ongoing investigation.

- Numerous risk and protective factors, including age, sex, genetics, and environmental and lifestyle factors, interact with pathophysiologic mechanisms in AD, but these should be understood to vary across diverse cultural groups, including different races and ethnicities.
- Biomarker and neuroimaging research has demonstrated how AD pathologic processes may lead to numerous cognitive and neuropsychiatric symptoms, such as impairments in memory, executive function, mood, and behavior.
- As the pathophysiology behind AD gains clarity, more potential treatment options are emerging, such as aducanumab, a monoclonal antibody directed against aggregated Aβ, which is the first novel medication approved for the treatment of AD in over 25 years.

DISCLOSURE

The authors have nothing to disclose. Support provided by the U.S. Department of Veterans Affairs (VA Career Development Award to Dr B.C. Yarns grant number IK2CX001884; VA Merit Review Award to Dr R.J. Melrose 5I01CX000409; Dr K.A. Holiday is supported by the VA Advanced Fellowship in Geriatrics).

REFERENCES

1. Alzheimer's Association. 2022 Alzheimer's disease facts and figures. Alzheimers Dement 2022;18(4):700–89.
2. American Psychiatric Association (APA). Diagnostic and statistical manual of mental disorders, fifth edition, text revision (DSM-5-TR). Arlington (VA): APA; 2022.
3. Lanctôt KL, Amatniek J, Ancoli-Israel S, et al. Neuropsychiatric signs and symptoms of Alzheimer's disease: New treatment paradigms. Alzheimers Dement 2017;3(3):440–9.
4. Khan S, Barve KH, Kumar MS. Recent Advancements in Pathogenesis, Diagnostics and Treatment of Alzheimer's Disease. Curr Neuropharmacol 2020; 18(11):1106–25.
5. Edwards FA. A Unifying Hypothesis for Alzheimer's Disease: From Plaques to Neurodegeneration. Trends Neurosci 2019;42(5):310–22.
6. Kumar K, Kumar A, Keegan RM, et al. Recent advances in the neurobiology and neuropharmacology of Alzheimer's disease. Biomed Pharmacother 2018;98: 297–307.
7. Kummer MP, Heneka MT. Truncated and modified amyloid-beta species. Alzheimers Res Ther 2014;6(3):28.
8. Martin L, Latypova X, Wilson CM, et al. Tau protein kinases: involvement in Alzheimer's disease. Ageing Res Rev 2013;12(1):289–309.
9. D'Amelio M, Rossini PM. Brain excitability and connectivity of neuronal assemblies in Alzheimer's disease: from animal models to human findings. Prog Neurobiol 2012;99(1):42–60.
10. Moossy J, Zubenko GS, Martinez AJ, et al. Bilateral symmetry of morphologic lesions in Alzheimer's disease. Arch Neurol 1988;45(3):251–4.
11. Snyder HM, Corriveau RA, Craft S, et al. Vascular contributions to cognitive impairment and dementia including Alzheimer's disease. Alzheimers Dement 2015;11(6):710–7.
12. Dodge HH, Zhu J, Woltjer R, et al. Risk of incident clinical diagnosis of Alzheimer's disease-type dementia attributable to pathology-confirmed vascular disease. Alzheimers Dement 2017;13(6):613–23.

13. Wolters FJ, Zonneveld HI, Hofman A, et al. Cerebral Perfusion and the Risk of Dementia: A Population-Based Study. Circulation 2017;136(8):719–28.

14. Hughes TM, Kuller LH, Barinas-Mitchell EJ, et al. Arterial stiffness and β-amyloid progression in nondemented elderly adults. JAMA Neurol 2014;71(5):562–8.

15. Hughes TM, Kuller LH, Barinas-Mitchell EJ, et al. Pulse wave velocity is associated with β-amyloid deposition in the brains of very elderly adults. Neurology 2013;81(19):1711–8.

16. Nation DA, Edmonds EC, Bangen KJ, et al. Pulse pressure in relation to tau-mediated neurodegeneration, cerebral amyloidosis, and progression to dementia in very old adults. JAMA Neurol 2015;72(5):546–53.

17. Wanleenuwat P, Iwanowski P, Kozubski W. Alzheimer's dementia: pathogenesis and impact of cardiovascular risk factors on cognitive decline. Postgrad Med 2019;131(7):415–22.

18. Rabin JS, Yang HS, Schultz AP, et al. Vascular risk and β-amyloid are synergistically associated with cortical tau. Ann Neurol 2019;85(2):272–9.

19. Bennett RE, Robbins AB, Hu M, et al. Tau induces blood vessel abnormalities and angiogenesis-related gene expression in P301L transgenic mice and human Alzheimer's disease. Proc Natl Acad Sci U S A 2018;115(6):E1289–98.

20. Chen ZR, Huang JB, Yang SL, et al. Role of Cholinergic Signaling in Alzheimer's Disease. Molecules 2022;27(6):1816.

21. Mufson EJ, Counts SE, Perez SE, et al. Cholinergic system during the progression of Alzheimer's disease: therapeutic implications. Expert Rev Neurother 2008;8(11):1703–18.

22. Hampel H, Mesulam MM, Cuello AC, et al. The cholinergic system in the pathophysiology and treatment of Alzheimer's disease. Brain 2018;141(7):1917–33.

23. Sultzer DL, Lim AC, Gordon HL, et al. Cholinergic receptor binding in unimpaired older adults, mild cognitive impairment, and Alzheimer's disease dementia. Alzheimers Res Ther 2022;14(1):25.

24. Sultzer DL, Melrose RJ, Riskin-Jones H, et al. Cholinergic Receptor Binding in Alzheimer Disease and Healthy Aging: Assessment In Vivo with Positron Emission Tomography Imaging. Am J Geriatr Psychiatry 2017;25(4):342–53.

25. Meltzer CC, Smith G, DeKosky ST, et al. Serotonin in aging, late-life depression, and Alzheimer's disease: the emerging role of functional imaging. Neuropsychopharmacology 1998;18(6):407–30.

26. Solas M, Van Dam D, Janssens J, et al. 5-HT(7) receptors in Alzheimer's disease. Neurochem Int 2021;150:105185.

27. Meneses A. 5-HT7 receptor stimulation and blockade: a therapeutic paradox about memory formation and amnesia. Front Behav Neurosci 2014;8:207.

28. Hu L, Wang B, Zhang Y. Serotonin 5-HT6 receptors affect cognition in a mouse model of Alzheimer's disease by regulating cilia function. Alzheimers Res Ther 2017;9(1):76.

29. Newcomer JW, Farber NB, Olney JW. NMDA receptor function, memory, and brain aging. Dialogues Clin Neurosci 2000;2(3):219–32.

30. Rudy CC, Hunsberger HC, Weitzner DS, et al. The role of the tripartite glutamatergic synapse in the pathophysiology of Alzheimer's disease. Aging Dis 2015; 6(2):131–48.

31. Olivares D, Deshpande VK, Shi Y, et al. N-methyl D-aspartate (NMDA) receptor antagonists and memantine treatment for Alzheimer's disease, vascular dementia and Parkinson's disease. Curr Alzheimer Res 2012;9(6):746–58.

32. Westbrook A, Braver TS. Dopamine Does Double Duty in Motivating Cognitive Effort. Neuron 2016;89(4):695–710.

33. Martorana A, Koch G. Is dopamine involved in Alzheimer's disease? Front Aging Neurosci 2014;6:252.

34. Robert PH, Mulin E, Malléa P, et al. REVIEW: Apathy diagnosis, assessment, and treatment in Alzheimer's disease. CNS Neurosci Ther 2010;16(5):263–71.

35. Pizzolato G, Chierichetti F, Fabbri M, et al. Reduced striatal dopamine receptors in Alzheimer's disease: single photon emission tomography study with the D2 tracer [123I]-IBZM. Neurology 1996;47(4):1065–8.

36. Solito E, Sastre M. Microglia function in Alzheimer's disease. Front Pharmacol 2012;3:14.

37. Calsolaro V, Edison P. Neuroinflammation in Alzheimer's disease: Current evidence and future directions. Alzheimers Dement 2016;12(6):719–32.

38. Mao P, Reddy PH. Aging and amyloid beta-induced oxidative DNA damage and mitochondrial dysfunction in Alzheimer's disease: implications for early intervention and therapeutics. Biochim Biophys Acta 2011;1812(11):1359–70.

39. Nikolac Perkovic M, Videtic Paska A, Konjevod M, et al. Epigenetics of Alzheimer's Disease. Biomolecules 2021;11(2):195.

40. Rosselli M, Uribe IV, Ahne E, et al. Culture, Ethnicity, and Level of Education in Alzheimer's Disease. Neurotherapeutics 2022;1–29.

41. Greenfield PM. You can't take it with you: Why ability assessments don't cross cultures. Am Psychol 1997;52(10):1115.

42. Vega IE, Cabrera LY, Wygant CM, et al. Alzheimer's disease in the Latino community: intersection of genetics and social determinants of health. J Alzheimers Dis 2017;58(4):979–92.

43. Lamar M, Barnes LL, Leurgans SE, et al. Acculturation in context: The relationship between acculturation and socioenvironmental factors with level of and change in cognition in older Latinos. J Gerontol B Psychol Sci Soc Sci 2021; 76(4):e129–39.

44. Barnes LL, Bennett DA. Alzheimer's disease in African Americans: risk factors and challenges for the future. Health Aff 2014;33(4):580–6.

45. Barnes LL, Wilson RS, Li Y, et al. Racial differences in the progression of cognitive decline in Alzheimer disease. Am J Geriatr Psychiatry 2005;13(11):959–67.

46. Weuve J, Rajan KB, Barnes LL, et al. Secular trends in cognitive performance in older black and white US adults, 1993–2012: Findings from the Chicago Health and Aging Project. J Gerontol B Psychol Sci Soc Sci 2018;73(suppl_1):S73–81.

47. Weiner MF. Perspective on race and ethnicity in Alzheimer's disease research. Alzheimers Dement 2008;4(4):233–8.

48. Schwartz BS, Glass TA, Bolla KI, et al. Disparities in cognitive functioning by race/ethnicity in the Baltimore Memory Study. Environ Health Perspect 2004; 112(3):314–20.

49. Armstrong RA. Risk factors for Alzheimer's disease. Folia Neuropathol 2019; 57(2):87–105.

50. Herrup K. Reimagining Alzheimer's disease—an age-based hypothesis. J Neurosci 2010;30(50):16755–62.

51. Trevisan K, Cristina-Pereira R, Silva-Amaral D, et al. Theories of Aging and the Prevalence of Alzheimer's Disease. Biomed Res Int 2019;2019:9171424.

52. Riedel BC, Thompson PM, Brinton RD. Age, APOE and sex: triad of risk of Alzheimer's disease. J Steroid Biochem Mol Biol 2016;160:134–47.

53. Farrer LA, Cupples LA, Haines JL, et al. Effects of age, sex, and ethnicity on the association between apolipoprotein E genotype and Alzheimer disease: a meta-analysis. JAMA 1997;278(16):1349–56.

54. Leduc V, Jasmin-Bélanger S, Poirier J. APOE and cholesterol homeostasis in Alzheimer's disease. Trends Mol Med 2010;16(10):469–77.
55. Reiman EM, Chen K, Liu X, et al. Fibrillar amyloid-β burden in cognitively normal people at 3 levels of genetic risk for Alzheimer's disease. Proc Natl Acad Sci U S A 2009;106(16):6820–5.
56. Castellano JM, Kim J, Stewart FR, et al. Human apoE isoforms differentially regulate brain amyloid-β peptide clearance. Sci Transl Med 2011;3(89). 89ra57.
57. Brookmeyer R, Gray S, Kawas C. Projections of Alzheimer's disease in the United States and the public health impact of delaying disease onset. Am J Public Health 1998;88(9):1337–42.
58. Fleisher A, Grundman M, Jack CR, et al. Sex, apolipoprotein E ε4 status, and hippocampal volume in mild cognitive impairment. Arch Neurol 2005;62(6): 953–7.
59. Perry DC, Sturm VE, Peterson MJ, et al. Association of traumatic brain injury with subsequent neurological and psychiatric disease: a meta-analysis. J Neurosurg 2016;124(2):511–26.
60. Schofield P, Tang M, Marder K, et al. Alzheimer's disease after remote head injury: an incidence study. J Neurol Neurosurg Psychiatry 1997;62(2):119–24.
61. Abner EL, Nelson PT, Schmitt FA, et al. Self-reported head injury and risk of late-life impairment and AD pathology in an AD center cohort. Dement Geriatr Cogn Disord 2014;37(5–6):294–306.
62. Tolppanen A-M, Taipale H, Hartikainen S. Head or brain injuries and Alzheimer's disease: A nested case-control register study. Dementia (London) 2017;13(12): 1371–9.
63. Barnes DE, Byers AL, Gardner RC, et al. Association of mild traumatic brain injury with and without loss of consciousness with dementia in US military veterans. JAMA Neurol 2018;75(9):1055–61.
64. Smith DH, Johnson VE, Stewart W. Chronic neuropathologies of single and repetitive TBI: substrates of dementia? Nat Rev Neurol 2013;9(4):211–21.
65. Mayeux R, Ottman R, Maestre G, et al. Synergistic effects of traumatic head injury and apolipoprotein-epsilon4 in patients with Alzheimer's disease. Neurology 1995;45(3):555–7.
66. Ramos-Cejudo J, Wisniewski T, Marmar C, et al. Traumatic brain injury and Alzheimer's disease: the cerebrovascular link. EBioMedicine 2018;28:21–30.
67. Xu X-J, Yang M-S, Zhang B, et al. Glucose metabolism: A link between traumatic brain injury and Alzheimer's disease. Chin J Traumatol 2021;24(01):5–10.
68. Bailey KC, Burmaster SA, Schaffert J, et al. Associations of Race-Ethnicity and History of Traumatic Brain Injury with Age at Onset of Alzheimer's Disease. J Neuropsychiatry Clin Neurosci 2020;32(3):280–5.
69. Huang C-H, Lin C-W, Lee Y-C, et al. Is traumatic brain injury a risk factor for neurodegeneration? A meta-analysis of population-based studies. BMC Neurol 2018;18(1):1–8.
70. Crane PK, Gibbons LE, Dams-O'Connor K, et al. Association of traumatic brain injury with late-life neurodegenerative conditions and neuropathologic findings. JAMA Neurol 2016;73(9):1062–9.
71. Dams-O'Connor K, Gibbons LE, Bowen JD, et al. Risk for late-life re-injury, dementia and death among individuals with traumatic brain injury: a population-based study. J Neurol Neurosurg Psychiatry 2013;84(2):177–82.
72. Gu D, Ou S, Liu G. Traumatic Brain Injury and Risk of Dementia and Alzheimer's Disease: A Systematic Review and Meta-Analysis. Neuroepidemiology 2022; 56(1):4–16.

73. Silva MVF, Loures CdMG, Alves LCV, et al. Alzheimer's disease: risk factors and potentially protective measures. J Biomed Sci 2019;26(1):1–11.

74. Killin LO, Starr JM, Shiue IJ, et al. Environmental risk factors for dementia: a systematic review. BMC Geriatr 2016;16(1):1–28.

75. Rizzi L, Rosset I, Roriz-Cruz M. Global epidemiology of dementia: Alzheimer's and vascular types. Biomed Res Int 2014;2014:908915.

76. Durazzo TC, Mattsson N, Weiner MW, Initiative AsDN. Smoking and increased Alzheimer's disease risk: a review of potential mechanisms. Dementia (London) 2014;10:S122–45.

77. Irwin MR, Vitiello MV. Implications of sleep disturbance and inflammation for Alzheimer's disease dementia. Lancet Neurol 2019;18(3):296–306.

78. Caruso A, Nicoletti F, Mango D, et al. Stress as risk factor for Alzheimer's disease. Pharmacol Res 2018;132:130–4.

79. Kline SA, Mega MS. Stress-induced neurodegeneration: the potential for coping as neuroprotective therapy. Am J Alzheimers Dis Other Demen 2020;35. 1533317520960873.

80. Livingston G, Sommerlad A, Orgeta V, et al. Dementia prevention, intervention, and care. Lancet 2017;390(10113):2673–734.

81. Nation DA, Hong S, Jak AJ, et al. Stress, exercise, and Alzheimer's disease: A neurovascular pathway. Med Hypotheses 2011;76(6):847–54.

82. Singh B, Parsaik AK, Mielke MM, et al. Association of mediterranean diet with mild cognitive impairment and Alzheimer's disease: a systematic review and meta-analysis. J Alzheimers Dis 2014;39(2):271–82.

83. Larsson SC, Traylor M, Malik R, et al. Modifiable pathways in Alzheimer's disease: Mendelian randomisation analysis. BMJ 2017;359:j5375.

84. Fritsch T, McClendon MJ, Smyth KA, et al. Effects of educational attainment on the clinical expression of Alzheimer's disease: results from a research registry. Am J Alzheimers Dis Other Demen 2001;16(6):369–76.

85. Stern Y. Cognitive reserve in ageing and Alzheimer's disease. Lancet Neurol 2012;11(11):1006–12.

86. Stern Y. What is cognitive reserve? Theory and research application of the reserve concept. J Int Neuropsychol Soc 2002;8(3):448–60.

87. Roth M, Tomlinson B, Blessed G. The relationship between quantitative measures of dementia and of degenerative changes in the cerebral grey matter of elderly subjects. Proc R Soc Med 1967;60(3):254.

88. Satz P. Brain reserve capacity on symptom onset after brain injury: a formulation and review of evidence for threshold theory. Neuropsychology 1993;7(3):273.

89. Avila JF, Rentería MA, Jones RN, et al. Education differentially contributes to cognitive reserve across racial/ethnic groups. Dementia (London) 2021;17(1): 70–80.

90. Bialystok E. Bilingualism: Pathway to cognitive reserve. Trends Cogn Sci 2021; 25(5):355–64.

91. Hort J, O'brien J, Gainotti G, et al. EFNS guidelines for the diagnosis and management of Alzheimer's disease. Eur J Neurol 2010;17(10):1236–48.

92. McKhann GM, Knopman DS, Chertkow H, et al. The diagnosis of dementia due to Alzheimer's disease: Recommendations from the National Institute on Aging-Alzheimer's Association workgroups on diagnostic guidelines for Alzheimer's disease. Dementia (London) 2011;7(3):263–9.

93. Peña-Casanova J, Sánchez-Benavides G, de Sola S, et al. Neuropsychology of Alzheimer's disease. Arch Med Res 2012;43(8):686–93.

94. Fama R, Sullivan EV, Shear PK, et al. Extent, pattern, and correlates of remote memory impairment in Alzheimer's disease and Parkinson's disease. Neuropsychology 2000;14(2):265.

95. Lezak M, Howieson D, Bigler E, et al. Neuropsychological assessment. New York: Oxford University Press; 2012.

96. Gross AL, Manly JJ, Pa J, et al. Cortical signatures of cognition and their relationship to Alzheimer's disease. Brain Imaging Behav 2012;6(4):584–98.

97. Insel PS, Mormino EC, Aisen PS, et al. Neuroanatomical spread of amyloid β and tau in Alzheimer's disease: implications for primary prevention. Brain Commun 2020;2(1):fcaa007.

98. Guarino A, Favieri F, Boncompagni I, et al. Executive functions in Alzheimer disease: a systematic review. Front Aging Neurosci 2019;10:437.

99. Woo CW, Koban L, Kross E, et al. Separate neural representations for physical pain and social rejection. Nat Commun 2014;5:5380.

100. Melrose RJ, Harwood D, Khoo T, et al. Association between cerebral metabolism and Rey–Osterrieth Complex Figure Test performance in Alzheimer's disease. J Clin Exp Neuropsychol 2013;35(3):246–58.

101. Bondi MW, Serody AB, Chan AS, et al. Cognitive and neuropathologic correlates of Stroop Color-Word Test performance in Alzheimer's disease. Neuropsychology 2002;16(3):335.

102. Ackley SF, Hayes-Larson E, Brenowitz WD, et al. Amyloid-PET imaging offers small improvements in predictions of future cognitive trajectories. Neuroimage Clin 2021;31:102713.

103. Bracco L, Bessi V, Piccini C, et al. Metabolic correlates of executive dysfunction. J Neurol 2007;254(8):1052–65.

104. Melrose RJ, Campa OM, Harwood DG, et al. The neural correlates of naming and fluency deficits in Alzheimer's disease: An FDG-PET study. Int J Geriatr Psychiatry 2009;24(8):885–93.

105. Apostolova LG, Lu P, Rogers S, et al. 3D mapping of language networks in clinical and pre-clinical Alzheimer's disease. Brain Lang 2008;104(1):33–41.

106. Grossman M, McMillan C, Moore P, et al. What's in a name: voxel-based morphometric analyses of MRI and naming difficulty in Alzheimer's disease, frontotemporal dementia and corticobasal degeneration. Brain 2004;127(3):628–49.

107. Henry JD, Crawford JR, Phillips LH. Verbal fluency performance in dementia of the Alzheimer's type: a meta-analysis. Neuropsychologia 2004;42(9):1212–22.

108. Mendez MF, Tomsak RL, Remler B. Disorders of the visual system in Alzheimer's disease. J Clin Neuroophthalmol 1990;10(1):62–9.

109. Cerquera-Jaramillo MA, Nava-Mesa MO, González-Reyes RE, et al. Visual features in Alzheimer's disease: from basic mechanisms to clinical overview. Neural Plast 2018;2018:2941783.

110. Lyketsos CG, Olin J. Depression in Alzheimer's disease: overview and treatment. Biol Psychiatry 2002;52(3):243–52.

111. Caraci F, Copani A, Nicoletti F, et al. Depression and Alzheimer's disease: neurobiological links and common pharmacological targets. Eur J Pharmacol 2010;626(1):64–71.

112. Starkstein SE, Jorge R, Mizrahi R, et al. A prospective longitudinal study of apathy in Alzheimer's disease. J Neurol Neurosurg Psychiatry 2006;77(1):8–11.

113. Johansson M, Stomrud E, Lindberg O, et al. Apathy and anxiety are early markers of Alzheimer's disease. Neurobiol Aging 2020;85:74–82.

114. Marshall GA, Fairbanks LA, Tekin S, et al. Neuropathologic correlates of apathy in Alzheimer's disease. Dement Geriatr Cogn Disord 2006;21(3):144–7.
115. Apostolova LG, Akopyan GG, Partiali N, et al. Structural correlates of apathy in Alzheimer's disease. Dement Geriatr Cogn Disord 2007;24(2):91–7.
116. Schneider LS, Dagerman KS. Psychosis of Alzheimer's disease: clinical characteristics and history. J Psychiatr Res 2004;38(1):105–11.
117. Koppel J, Sunday S, Goldberg TE, et al. Psychosis in Alzheimer's disease is associated with frontal metabolic impairment and accelerated decline in working memory: findings from the Alzheimer's Disease Neuroimaging Initiative. Am J Geriatr Psychiatry 2014;22(7):698–707.
118. Lanctôt KL, Herrmann N, Eryavec G, et al. Central serotonergic activity is related to the aggressive behaviors of Alzheimer's disease. Neuropsychopharmacology 2002;27(4):646–54.
119. Tekin S, Mega MS, Masterman DM, et al. Orbitofrontal and anterior cingulate cortex neurofibrillary tangle burden is associated with agitation in Alzheimer disease. Ann Neurol 2001;49(3):355–61.
120. Giacobini E, Cuello AC, Fisher A. Reimagining cholinergic therapy for Alzheimer's disease. Brain 2022. https://doi.org/10.1093/brain/awac096.
121. Mukhopadhyay S, Banerjee D. A Primer on the Evolution of Aducanumab: The First Antibody Approved for Treatment of Alzheimer's Disease. J Alzheimers Dis 2021;83(4):1537–52.
122. Jeremic D, Jiménez-Díaz L, Navarro-López JD. Past, present and future of therapeutic strategies against amyloid-β peptides in Alzheimer's disease: a systematic review. Ageing Res Rev 2021;72:101496.
123. Livingston G, Huntley J, Sommerlad A, et al. Dementia prevention, intervention, and care: 2020 report of the Lancet Commission. Lancet 2020;396(10248):413–46.
124. Cummings JL, Tong G, Ballard C. Treatment Combinations for Alzheimer's Disease: Current and Future Pharmacotherapy Options. J Alzheimers Dis 2019;67(3):779–94.

Epidemiology and Risk Factors for Dementia

Christina S. Dintica, PhD[a], Kristine Yaffe, MD[a,b,*]

KEYWORDS

- Dementia • Aging • Epidemiology • Cognition

KEY POINTS

- The prevalence of all-cause dementia increases sharply with age and is expected to triple in the next 50 years.
- Up until recently, there has been little progress in dementia drug development, and even now, drug efficacy remains controversial.
- Evidence suggests that there are factors that increase the risk of dementia, many of which are modifiable and may play an important role in prevention.
- Multidomain interventions targeting several of these risk factors are a promising avenue for dementia prevention.

INTRODUCTION

Dementia is a syndrome characterized by cognitive decline and functional impairment that encompasses many different specific diseases. Alzheimer's disease (AD) is the most common type of dementia, accounting for approximately 60% of dementia cases (either alone or in combination); vascular dementia (VaD) accounts for another 10% to 20% with other dementia types such as frontotemporal degeneration and Lewy body dementia accounting for the remainder. To date, most epidemiologic research on dementia has examined the prevalence, incidence, and risk factors for either all-cause dementia or AD. Therefore, in this review, the authors also discuss primarily what is known about the epidemiology of all-cause dementia and AD, about other specific dementias when data are available.

THE IMPENDING PUBLIC HEALTH CRISIS OF DEMENTIA
Prevalence and Incidence

The prevalence of all-cause dementia, as well as for AD and VaD, increases sharply with age. For AD alone, the prevalence may be as high as 11% in US adults over

[a] Department of Psychiatry and Behavioral Sciences, University of California, San Francisco, San Francisco, CA, USA; [b] San Francisco VA Health Care System, San Francisco, CA, USA
* Corresponding author. Department of Psychiatry, University of California, San Francisco, 675 18th Street, San Francisco, CA 94143.
E-mail address: kristine.yaffe@ucsf.edu

Psychiatr Clin N Am 45 (2022) 677–689
https://doi.org/10.1016/j.psc.2022.07.011
0193-953X/22/© 2022 Elsevier Inc. All rights reserved.

the age of 65 years and nearly 32% in adults over the age of 85 years.[1] In 2013, there were approximately 5 million people in the United States with dementia. It is estimated that this number will nearly triple to 13.2 million by 2050.[1] The incidence of all-cause dementia, as well as AD and VaD, also rises exponentially with age. Interestingly, several reports have described temporal trends indicating declines in dementia incidence within study cohorts over several decades.[2,3] Such findings, while not universal, have been attributed to society-level changes such as increased education and improved health care; however, the reasons behind this improvement have not clearly been understood to date.

The Potential for Prevention

Given the dramatic increases that are expected in both the prevalence and costs of AD and other dementias, it is critical to identify factors that are associated with increased disease risk and to develop successful prevention and treatment strategies. Because most dementias occur most commonly in very old age, interventions that delay the onset of disease have the potential to reduce prevalence dramatically over time. It has been suggested that a 10% to 25% reduction in seven modifiable risk factors of AD could prevent as many as 1.1 to 3.0 million AD cases worldwide and 184,000 to 492,000 cases in the United States.[4] These risk factors are modifiable and targetable by intervention.[5] Strategies focusing on several modifiable risk factors for dementia may be promising alternatives; they can also help in identifying effective preventive strategies.

Two large reports have summarized the current evidence on preventative strategies for dementia. The National Academy of Medicine report summarized findings from interventions for preventing dementia or mild cognitive impairment (MCI) based on findings from large randomized clinical trials (>250 participants per arm), with at least 6 months of follow-up.[6] The conclusion of the report was that the available evidence from large randomized trials remains inconclusive, and therefore, there are no specific interventions with strong enough evidence to warrant a public health advice for the prevention of dementia. Nevertheless, the National Academy of Medicine report found promising evidence of the potential benefit of three types of intervention: cognitive training, blood pressure management in people with hypertension, and physical activity. Moreover, the report highlighted that there are substantial challenges in conducting randomized trials of interventions for dementia, which has a long latency period and, until recently, have had limited consensus on biomarkers.

In contrast, the Lancet review of evidence covered both observational studies and randomized trials with no defined evaluation of evidence. The Lancet commission concluded that 40% of dementia could be prevented by modifying 12 risk factors: low education, midlife hearing loss, obesity, and hypertension, late-life depression, smoking, physical inactivity, diabetes, social isolation, traumatic brain injury (TBI), alcohol consumption, and pollution.[7] The recommendations of the report are mainly based on the estimation of population attributable risk for these factors. Furthermore, the report emphasizes the life course conceptual framework in which risk factors and modification of their risk exert influence decades before clinical disease onset.

The question is how can the available evidence be used to inform clinical practice? One alternative is to encourage patients, based on modestly strong evidence, to be physically and cognitively active and to manage cardiovascular risk factors. The other option is to make overall recommendations for improved health which may benefit brain health as well. More precise and "person-centered" recommendations will require more evidence. The authors summarize the most promising avenues for dementia prevention as follows.

RISK FACTORS FOR DEMENTIA
Sociodemographic Risk Factors

Race

Racial and ethnic disparities in dementia incidence are well-documented in the United States. Of note, several studies have found that the incidence of dementia and AD is approximately two times higher in Blacks and Hispanics compared with Whites.[8,9] Findings from a large sample from an integrated health care system with equal access to health care followed for 14 years suggest that dementia incidence was highest among African Americans and American Indian/Alaska Native, lowest among Asian Americans, and intermediate among Latinos, Pacific Islanders, and Whites.[10] These results suggest that efforts aimed at reducing such disparities may affect the incidence of dementia in ethnic/race minorities. For instance, findings from Weuve and colleagues[11] suggest that persistent racial differences in cognitive level—rather than differences in cognitive decline in old age—likely underlie the higher risk of incident dementia among Blacks. Findings from the Health ABC study suggest that differences in the burden of risk factors, especially socioeconomic status, may contribute to the higher rates of dementia seen among Black compared with White older people.[12] Hence, higher dementia incidence in ethnic/race minorities could reflect differences in cognitive reserve caused by racial disparities over the lifespan in, for example, education, access to material and social resources, resources including health care, and exposure to discrimination.[13,14] A recent large study from the Veterans Health System reported greater dementia incidence among Black and Hispanic older veterans even after accounting for several psychiatric and comorbidities.[15] Additional research is needed to determine what underlies these health disparities and to develop interventions that target those at highest risk.

Education

There is considerable evidence that older adults with greater education are less likely to develop dementia.[16,17] One highly cited study found that nuns with high idea density and grammatical complexity early in life were less likely to develop dementia later in life.[18] This may reflect, in part, a measurement bias, in which older adults with more education or higher intelligence perform better on cognitive tests, making dementia more difficult to detect. However, there is growing evidence that education may be associated with greater cognitive or neuronal reserves, which may protect against or minimize the impact of neurodegenerative disorders.[19] A recent study suggests that education is positively associated with cognitive ability in early life, before reaching a plateau in late adolescence, when brain reaches greatest plasticity, with relatively few further gains with education after age 20 years.[20] This suggests that education increases the overall level of cognition, leaving more "reserve" for decline to occur before becoming clinically significant.

Cardiovascular Risk Factors

Traditionally, AD has been viewed as a neurodegenerative disorder distinct from VaD. However, autopsy studies have suggested that many patients with clinical AD also have evidence of vascular pathology,[21] especially with increasing age. There also is growing evidence that risk factors for cardiovascular disease (CVD), such as diabetes mellitus, obesity, hypertension, and hyperlipidemia, are associated with a higher risk of developing AD and other dementias. Treatment and management of cardiovascular risk factors has thus far shown the most benefit in lowering the risk of dementia, particularly VaD.

Diabetes

Population-based, longitudinal studies have consistently found that older adults with diabetes experienced approximately a twofold increase in dementia risk.[22,23] When specific dementia subtypes are examined, diabetes is associated more strongly with VaD than AD.[24] Findings have also suggested that hypoglycemia, which commonly occurs in subjects with diabetes, is associated with a twofold increased risk of developing dementia,[25] suggesting caution in being too aggressive with treatment of diabetes in older adults. In a recent systematic review and meta-analysis, diabetes conferred a 1.25- to 1.91-fold excess risk for cognitive disorders (cognitive impairment and dementia). However, the use of antidiabetic medication reduced the risk of dementia by 47%.[26] Finally, pilot trials of intranasal insulin have shown positive effects on cognitive performance.[27,28]

Hypertension

A recent review concluded that hypertension in midlife, especially if not treated effectively, is associated with an increased risk of dementia and AD in late life.[29] Pooled analysis showed that high blood pressure in midlife was associated with 60% increased risk of dementia.[4] In late life, both very high systolic blood pressure and very low diastolic blood pressure have been associated with an increased risk of dementia.[30] It has been proposed that high blood pressure may lead to dementia by increasing the risk of small vessel ischemia and stroke as well as increasing neurodegeneration, whereas low blood pressure in late life may lead to dementia by increasing the risk of cerebral hypoperfusion and hypoxia. A review of randomized controlled trials examining the efficacy of antihypertensive treatment in preventing cognitive impairment and dementia in older adults did not find strong evidence.[31] In the more recent SPRINT-MIND trial in adults with hypertension, more aggressive systolic blood pressure treatment reduced the risk of dementia and MCI.[32]

High cholesterol

There is increasing evidence from observational epidemiologic cohorts that having high cholesterol levels is associated with an increased risk of dementia.[33] High cholesterol, which is linked to risk of atherosclerosis and cerebrovascular disease,[34] has been linked to cortical infarcts and white matter lesions.[35] In particular, studies on the role of total cholesterol at midlife have almost consistently found that higher levels of cholesterol are associated with dementia.[36] On the contrary, evidence on the role of late-life cholesterol on dementia and cognitive health has been inconsistent and reported either no associations or associations in the opposite direction to those observed using midlife cholesterol.[37] Preventive efforts have focused on the potential protective role of statins on dementia. Although some evidence indicates that statins are protective against dementia and cognitive impairment,[38,39] no randomized clinical trials have clearly shown evidence of either positive or negative effect of statins on cognition.[40] Moreover, the US Food and Drug Administration has issued a safety warning regarding potential memory loss associated with statin use although this has not been well-documented.[40]

Obesity

According to a recent review, the role of obesity in cognitive decline and AD pathology remains relatively unclear.[41] Some studies have shown no association, whereas others have shown an inverse or U-shaped association. Studies have shown that the risk of developing dementia may differ according to the timing of obesity, that is, higher in midlife versus lower in late life.[42,43] Findings from the Whitehall study showed that obesity at age 50 years but not at 60 or 70 years was associated with a higher risk of dementia.[44] Findings of protective effects of obesity or overweight on dementia risk in older groups may reflect biases, especially weight loss during the pre-clinical phase before dementia diagnosis. Epidemiologic evidence on the association between obesity and risk of dementia may partly reflect the role of obesity as a marker of vascular and inflammatory damage.[45]

Multiple cardiovascular risk factors

Several studies have evaluated the effects of multiple or composite cardiovascular risk factors on the risk of dementia. Among members of a large health-maintenance orga-nization, subjects who had diabetes, hypertension, and high cholesterol or were smokers at midlife were more likely to develop dementia later in life, and the effects of each factor were approximately additive.[43] Similarly, the "metabolic syndrome" (MetS), which is a clustering of cardiovascular disorders, has been associated with an increased risk of dementia,[46] cognitive impairment, and cognitive decline, espe-cially in older adults with high levels of inflammation.[47] Findings from the Framingham study showed that both midlife and late-life MetS were associated with lower level of cognitive functioning but not cognitive trajectories.[48] Studies using composites of vascular risk scores showed that ideal cardiovascular health, defined by guidelines by the American Heart Association, in young adulthood and its maintenance to middle age is associated with better psychomotor speed, executive function, and verbal memory in midlife.[49]

Behavioral Factors

Cognitive, social, and physical activity

There is growing evidence that mental or cognitive activity may help older adults to build or maintain a reserve that may delay the onset of overt dementia symptoms.[50] Several observational studies found that older adults who engage in mentally stimu-lating activities, such as reading or playing games, are at lower risk of developing cognitive decline and dementia.[51] In midlife, engaging such activities was associated with maintaining cognition, independent of education, occupation, late-life activities, and current structural brain health.[52] However, a recent study showed that partici-pants who had a decline in leisure activity over the study period had a higher dementia risk compared with participants who had continuously lower engagement,[53] suggest-ing that the reduction and withdrawal from cognitively stimulating activity may reflect prodromal dementia.

Similar to the evidence of mental activity, staying socially active may reduce the risk of AD and other dementias.[54,55] In a longitudinal study of older adults, those who had engaged in social activities were less likely to develop dementia during follow-up.[56] Some have proposed that social activities might reduce the risk of dementia through mechanisms such as increasing cognitive reserve, reducing vascular disease, and the glucocorticoid cascade.[57] However, an analysis in the Honolulu-Asia Aging Study suggesting that low social engagement in late life might also reflect prodromal dementia.[54]

Several lines of evidence suggest that physical activity may protect against cogni-tive decline and dementia in older adults. In a study of almost 6000 older women, those in the highest quartile of blocks walked per week were less likely to experience substantial cognitive decline compared with those in the lowest quartile.[58] A recent systematic review of prospective studies and intervention studies in older adults found that physical activity was inversely associated with the risk of dementia in most studies.[59] However, findings from randomized trials have been mixed; one trial showed that among sedentary older adults with no cognitive impairment, a 24-month moderate-intensity physical activity program compared with a health education program did not result in improvements in cognitive function,[60] whereas others reported that both aerobic exercise and resistance training result in cognitive benefit.[61] Current evidence does not allow drawing specific practical recommendations concerning the types, frequency, intensity, or duration of physical activity that may be protective against dementia. Nevertheless, physical activity has proven to have health benefits for the brain.

Alcohol consumption

A meta-analysis of epidemiologic studies found that alcohol use was associated with decreased risk of any dementia.[62] Several studies have found that light-to-moderate drinkers have a 30% to 50% reduction in the risk of dementia compared with non-drinkers.[63,64] A recent study involving female veterans found that alcohol use disorder among female US veterans aged more than 55 years seems to be associated with a more than threefold increase of dementia.[65] In several countries, guidelines define thresholds for harmful alcohol consumption much higher than 14 units/wk. The above findings encourage the downward revision of such guidelines to promote cognitive health at older ages.

Neuropsychiatric Factors

Depression

Several longitudinal studies have found that older people with depressive symptoms have an increased risk of cognitive decline and approximately a twofold increase in dementia incidence,[66,67] whereas others have found that depressive symptoms seem to coincide with[68] or follow[69] dementia onset rather than precede it. In a longitudinal study of almost 6000 older women, a long-term cumulative depressive symptoms burden over nearly 20 years was strongly and independently associated with greater cognitive decline and higher odds of developing dementia and MCI.[70] More studies are needed to disentangle the directionality of these associations. Additional research is needed to determine whether treatment of depressive symptoms may reduce the risk of dementia.

Traumatic brain injury

Head injury with loss of consciousness was one of the earliest factors to be associated with an increased risk of dementia and AD.[71] Two studies, including a recent analysis of nearly 1 million US veterans aged 55 years or older, having TBI was associated with a threefold increased risk of developing dementia.[72] Importantly, even mild TBI without loss of consciousness has associated with more than a twofold increase in the risk of dementia diagnosis.[73] However, other longitudinal studies found no significant association between head injury and risk of AD or dementia.[74,75] Further work is warranted especially with neuropathology and neuroimaging to elucidate the mechanisms for this association.

Sleep

One of the most promising avenues of research in the epidemiology of dementia is the relationship between sleep and cognitive health. Patients with dementia frequently experience sleep disturbances, including insomnia, poor sleep quality, excessive daytime sleepiness, and disrupted circadian rhythms.[76] Growing evidence suggested that as much as 50% to 80% increased risk of dementia is associated with sleep disturbances, including insomnia, sleep-disordered breathing, disrupted circadian rhythms, and sleep-related movement disorders.[77–80] Several studies have found a U-shaped association between sleep duration and risk of dementia,[81,82] indicating negative effects of both short and long sleep duration. Given that current evidence indicates a bidirectional relationship between sleep disturbances and dementia, sleep interventions are underway to examine their use of prevention and treatment of dementia. Future research is needed to test whether sleep disturbances could be the risk factors for dementia and to explore the use of sleep interventions in patients at high risk for dementia.[83]

MULTIDOMAIN INTERVENTIONS

The etiology of dementia is multifactorial and consequently has several potentially modifiable risk factors and protective factors. Therefore, there has been a shift in recent years from single-domain interventions such as diet or exercise toward multidomain interventions for dementia prevention, targeting several modifiable risk factors.

The French Multidomain Alzheimer Preventive Trial was one of the first multidomain lifestyle interventions, composing of cognitive training and advice on nutrition and physical activity in participants 70 years or older.[84] Positive effects were reported among individuals with an increased risk of dementia, defined as a Cardiovascular Risk Factors, Aging and Dementia (CAIDE) score ≥ 6 or the presence of amyloid-β on PET imaging.[84] The Dutch Prevention of Dementia by Intensive Vascular Care trial was a cardiovascular intervention spanning 6 years for the prevention of dementia in participants aged 70 to 78 years.[85] The protective effects of dementia were reported in a subgroup of participants with baseline untreated hypertension, for whom therapy was initiated through the intervention.[85] In the FINGER trial, a multidomain approach including diet, exercise, cognitive training, and vascular risk monitoring was implemented to prevent cognitive decline in at-risk older adults from the general population. Compared with the control group that received general health advice, the intervention group improved approximately 25% more on a neuropsychological test battery.[86]

To date, there has not been a completed multidomain Alzheimer's risk reduction trial in the United States. The previous multidomain risk reduction trials have generally involved intensive interventions which may be difficult to implement within a real-world setting. To address this, the Systematic Multidomain Alzheimer's Risk Reduction Trial was developed and is currently underway.[87] This is a randomized pilot trial testing a personalized, pragmatic, multidomain intervention within the US integrated health care delivery system, with the primary aim of AD risk reduction.[87] The larger US Pointer, modeled after the FINGER trial, is also underway. The results from multidomain trials have been mixed; however, there is evidence of benefit in adults with vascular risk factors.

SUMMARY AND FUTURE DIRECTIONS

As described above, dementia is a multifactorial disorder. Several large, prospective, observational studies have identified a variety of factors that may prevent or delay onset of dementia. These include sociodemographic, cardiovascular, behavioral, and neuropsychiatric risk factors. However, the evidence base to date is lacking in certain respects, reflected in that intervention trials have often yielded conflicting results. One aspect where efforts should be increased is the diversity of study populations and recruitment of observational studies and intervention trials. Recruiting study populations that better reflect the distributions of race, ethnicity, education, and socioeconomic status in the general population would help ensure the generalizability of clinical trial results to traditionally underrepresented populations.

Another aspect that needs more consideration is that several risk factors are age-dependent and their association with dementia differs across the life course (midlife vs later life). Randomized controlled trials of some pharmacologic interventions targeting these risk factors, such as antihypertensive medications, have shown promising results, whereas others, such as cholesterol-lowering medications, have yielded disappointing or inconclusive results. The timing of an intervention relative to the onset of pathophysiological changes can have a large impact on the likelihood of observing a benefit. Therefore, to better understand the epidemiology of dementia and the potential of interventions at specific time windows, future studies need to address the life course and long preclinical aspects of this disorder.

Having more inclusive clinical trials and more attention to timing of interventions are crucial to synthesize evidence to guide clinicians and policy makers to prevent or delay dementia. There are established evidence-based national campaigns for the prevention and treatment of heart disease and stroke. Similar national campaigns are needed to inform the public that dementia risk is also susceptible to the effects of many cardiovascular risk factors and may eventually include other proven lifestyle or risk-reduction strategies as discussed in this review. Given the burden of dementia today, even relatively small reductions in dementia incidence would have a dramatic public health impact. The goal is that similar to other diseases such as CVD, dementia could be tackled by both prevention and treatment options. Studying the effects of drugs and prevention together will be the best strategy moving forward in dementia management.

CLINICS CARE POINTS

- In patients with cardiovascular disease or vascular risk factors such as hypertension and diabetes, treatments of these conditions may reduce the risk of dementia.
- Patients with neuropsychiatric conditions such as TBI, Post-traumatic stress disorder (PTSD), or depression may be more vulnerable to cognitive decline which should be monitored closely.
- The life period of certain risk factors is important to consider, some may confer more risk in midlife, and may not contribute much to risk in late life.

ACKNOWLEDGEMENT

This work was also supported by NIA R35AG071916 (Yaffe) and an Alzheimer's Association grant AARF-21-851960 (Dintica).

DISCLOSURE

The authors have nothing to disclose.

REFERENCES

1. Hebert LE, Weuve J, Scherr PA, et al. Alzheimer disease in the United States (2010-2050) estimated using the 2010 census. Neurology 2013;80(19):1778–83.
2. Wu Y-T, Beiser AS, Breteler MMB, et al. The changing prevalence and incidence of dementia over time — current evidence. Nat Rev Neurol 2017;13(6):327–39.
3. Gao S, Burney HN, Callahan CM, et al. Incidence of dementia and alzheimer disease over time: a meta-analysis. J Am Geriatr Soc 2019;67(7):1361–9.

4. Barnes DE, Yaffe K. The projected effect of risk factor reduction on Alzheimer's disease prevalence. Lancet Neurol 2011;10(9):819–28.

5. Livingston G, Sommerlad A, Orgeta V, et al. Dementia prevention, intervention, and care. Lancet 2017;(17):6736. https://doi.org/10.1016/S0140-6736(17)31363-6.

6. Leshner AI, Landis S, Stroud C, et al. Preventing cognitive decline and dementia. In: Leshner AI, Landis S, Stroud C, Downey A, editors. Washington (D.C): National Academies Press; 2017. https://doi.org/10.17226/24782.

7. Livingston G, Huntley J, Sommerlad A, et al. Dementia prevention, intervention, and care: 2020 report of the Lancet Commission. Lancet 2020;396(10248):413–46.

8. Folstein MF, Bassett SS, Anthony JC, et al. Dementia: Case Ascertainment in a Community Survey. J Gerontol 1991;46(4):M132–8.

9. Tang M-X, Cross P, Andrews H, et al. Incidence of AD in African-Americans, Caribbean Hispanics, and Caucasians in northern Manhattan. Neurology 2001;56(1):49–56.

10. Mayeda ER, Glymour MM, Quesenberry CP, et al. Inequalities in dementia incidence between six racial and ethnic groups over 14 years. Alzheimer's Dement 2016;12(3):216–24.

11. Weuve J, Barnes LL, Mendes de Leon CF, et al. Cognitive Aging in Black and White Americans. Epidemiology 2018;29(1):151–9.

12. Yaffe K, Falvey C, Harris TB, et al. Effect of socioeconomic disparities on incidence of dementia among biracial older adults: prospective study. BMJ 2013;347(dec19 5):f7051.

13. Bell ML, Ebisu K. Environmental inequality in exposures to airborne particulate matter components in the United States. Environ Health Perspect 2012;120(12):1699–704.

14. Caunca MR, Odden MC, Glymour MM, et al. Association of racial residential segregation throughout young adulthood and cognitive performance in middle-aged participants in the CARDIA Study. JAMA Neurol 2020;77(8):1000.

15. Kornblith E, Bahorik A, Boscardin WJ, et al. Association of race and ethnicity with incidence of dementia among older adults. JAMA 2022;327(15):1488–95.

16. Foubert-Samier A, Catheline G, Amieva H, et al. Education, occupation, leisure activities, and brain reserve: a population-based study. Neurobiol Aging 2012;33(2):423.e15–25.

17. Gross AL, Mungas DM, Crane PK, et al. Effects of education and race on cognitive decline: an integrative study of generalizability versus study-specific results. Psychol Aging 2015;30(4):863–80.

18. Snowdon DA, Kemper SJ, Mortimer JA, et al. Linguistic ability in early life and cognitive function and Alzheimer's disease in late life. Findings from the Nun Study. JAMA 1996;275(7):528–32.

19. Jones RN, Manly J, Glymour MM, et al. Conceptual and Measurement Challenges in Research on Cognitive Reserve. J Int Neuropsychol Soc 2011;17(4):593–601.

20. Kremen WS, Beck A, Elman JA, et al. Influence of young adult cognitive ability and additional education on later-life cognition. Proc Natl Acad Sci 2019;116(6):2021–6.

21. Snowdon DA, Greiner LH, Mortimer JA, et al. Brain infarction and the clinical expression of Alzheimer disease. The Nun Study. JAMA 1997;277(10):813–7.

22. Ahtiluoto S, Polvikoski T, Peltonen M, et al. Diabetes, Alzheimer disease, and vascular dementia: a population-based neuropathologic study. Neurology 2010;75(13):1195–202.

23. Hassing LB, Johansson B, Nilsson SE, et al. Diabetes Mellitus Is a Risk Factor for Vascular Dementia, but Not for Alzheimer's Disease: A Population-Based Study of the Oldest Old. Int Psychogeriatrics 2002;14(3):239–48.

24. Areosa Sastre A, Vernooij RW, González-Colaço Harmand M, et al. Effect of the treatment of Type 2 diabetes mellitus on the development of cognitive impairment and dementia. Cochrane Database Syst Rev 2017. https://doi.org/10.1002/14651858.CD003804.pub2.

25. Yaffe K. Association Between Hypoglycemia and Dementia in a Biracial Cohort of Older Adults With Diabetes Mellitus. JAMA Intern Med 2013;173(14):1300.

26. Xue M, Xu W, Ou Y-N, et al. Diabetes mellitus and risks of cognitive impairment and dementia: a systematic review and meta-analysis of 144 prospective studies. Ageing Res Rev 2019;55:100944.

27. Craft S. Intranasal insulin therapy for alzheimer disease and amnestic mild cognitive impairment. Arch Neurol 2012;69(1):29.

28. Hallschmid M. Intranasal Insulin for Alzheimer's Disease. CNS Drugs 2021;35(1):21–37.

29. Qiu C. Preventing Alzheimer's disease by targeting vascular risk factors: hope and gap. In: de la Torre J, editor. J Alzheimer's Dis 2012;32(3):721–31.

30. Qiu C, Winblad B, Fratiglioni L. The age-dependent relation of blood pressure to cognitive function and dementia. Lancet Neurol 2005;4(8):487–99.

31. McGuinness B, Todd S, Passmore P, et al. Blood pressure lowering in patients without prior cerebrovascular disease for prevention of cognitive impairment and dementia. Cochrane Database Syst Rev 2009. https://doi.org/10.1002/14651858.CD004034.pub3.

32. Williamson JD, Pajewski NM, Auchus AP, et al. Effect of intensive vs standard blood pressure control on probable dementia. JAMA 2019;321(6):553.

33. Shepardson NE. Cholesterol Level and Statin Use in Alzheimer Disease. Arch Neurol 2011;68(10):1239.

34. Launer LJ, White LR, Petrovitch H, et al. Cholesterol and neuropathologic markers of AD: a population-based autopsy study. Neurology 2001;57(8):1447–52.

35. Amarenco P, Labreuche J, Elbaz A, et al. Blood Lipids in Brain Infarction Subtypes. Cerebrovasc Dis 2006;22(2–3):101–8.

36. Anstey KJ, Ashby-Mitchell K, Peters R. Updating the Evidence on the Association between Serum Cholesterol and Risk of Late-Life Dementia: Review and Meta-Analysis. J Alzheimer's Dis 2017;56(1):215–28.

37. Reitz C, Tang M-X, Schupf N, et al. Association of Higher Levels of High-Density Lipoprotein Cholesterol in Elderly Individuals and Lower Risk of Late-Onset Alzheimer Disease. Arch Neurol 2010;67(12). https://doi.org/10.1001/archneurol.2010.297.

38. Beydoun MA, Beason-Held LL, Kitner-Triolo MH, et al. Statins and serum cholesterol's associations with incident dementia and mild cognitive impairment. J Epidemiol Community Heal 2011;65(11):949–57.

39. Dufouil C, Richard F, Fievet N, et al. APOE genotype, cholesterol level, lipid-lowering treatment, and dementia: The Three-City Study. Neurology 2005;64(9):1531–8.

40. Padala KP, Padala PR, Potter JF. Statins: a case for drug withdrawal in patients with dementia. J Am Geriatr Soc 2010;58(6):1214–6.

41. Hildreth KL, Pelt RE, Schwartz RS. Obesity, Insulin Resistance, and Alzheimer's Disease. Obesity 2012;20(8):1549–57.

42. Anstey KJ, Cherbuin N, Budge M, et al. Body mass index in midlife and late-life as a risk factor for dementia: a meta-analysis of prospective studies. Obes Rev 2011;12(5):e426–37.

43. Whitmer RA, Sidney S, Selby J, et al. Midlife cardiovascular risk factors and risk of dementia in late life. Neurology 2005;64(2):277–81.

44. Kivimäki M, Luukkonen R, Batty GD, et al. Body mass index and risk of dementia: Analysis of individual-level data from 1.3 million individuals. Alzheimer's Dement 2018;14(5):601–9.

45. Zeki Al Hazzouri A, Stone KL, Haan MN, et al. Mild Cognitive Impairment, and Dementia Among Elderly Women. Journals Gerontol Ser A Biol Sci Med Sci 2013; 68(2):175–80.

46. Reitz C, Brayne C, Mayeux R. Epidemiology of Alzheimer disease. Nat Rev Neurol 2011;7(3):137–52.

47. Yaffe K. The metabolic syndrome, inflammation, and risk of cognitive decline. JAMA 2004;292(18):2237.

48. Bangen KJ, Armstrong NM, Au R, et al. In: Brandt J, editor. Metabolic syndrome and cognitive trajectories in the framingham offspring study. J Alzheimer's dis, 71. 2019. p. 931–43 (3).

49. Reis JP, Loria CM, Launer LJ, et al. Cardiovascular health through young adulthood and cognitive functioning in midlife. Ann Neurol 2013;73(2):170–9.

50. Stern Y. What is cognitive reserve? Theory and research application of the reserve concept. J Int Neuropsychol Soc 2002;8(3):448–60.

51. Treiber KA, Carlson MC, Corcoran C, et al. Cognitive stimulation and cognitive and functional decline in Alzheimer's disease: the Cache County Dementia Progression Study. Journals Gerontol Ser B Psychol Sci Soc Sci 2011;66B(4): 416–25.

52. Chan D, Shafto M, Kievit R, et al. Lifestyle activities in mid-life contribute to cognitive reserve in late-life, independent of education, occupation, and late-life activities. Neurobiol Aging 2018;70:180–3.

53. Sommerlad A, Sabia S, Livingston G, et al. Leisure activity participation and risk of dementia. Neurology 2020;95(20):e2803–15.

54. Saczynski JS, Pfeifer LA, Masaki K, et al. The Effect of Social Engagement on Incident Dementia. Am J Epidemiol 2006;163(5):433–40.

55. Sharp ES, Reynolds CA, Pedersen NL, et al. Cognitive engagement and cognitive aging: Is openness protective? Psychol Aging 2010;25(1):60–73.

56. Scarmeas N, Levy G, Tang M-X, et al. Influence of leisure activity on the incidence of Alzheimer's Disease. Neurology 2001;57(12):2236–42.

57. Fratiglioni L, Paillard-Borg S, Winblad B. An active and socially integrated lifestyle in late life might protect against dementia. Lancet Neurol 2004;3(6):343–53.

58. Yaffe K, Barnes D, Nevitt M, et al. A Prospective Study of Physical Activity and Cognitive Decline in Elderly Women. Arch Intern Med 2001;161(14):1703.

59. Stephen R, Hongisto K, Solomon A, et al. Physical Activity and Alzheimer's Disease: A Systematic Review. Journals Gerontol Ser A Biol Sci Med Sci 2017;glw251. https://doi.org/10.1093/gerona/glw251.

60. Sink KM, Espeland MA, Castro CM, et al. Effect of a 24-Month Physical Activity Intervention vs Health Education on Cognitive Outcomes in Sedentary Older Adults. JAMA 2015;314(8):781.

61. Smith PJ, Blumenthal JA, Hoffman BM, et al. Aerobic exercise and neurocognitive performance: a meta-analytic review of randomized controlled trials. Psychosom Med 2010;72(3):239–52.

62. Anstey KJ, Mack HA, Cherbuin N. Alcohol consumption as a risk factor for dementia and cognitive decline: meta-analysis of prospective studies. Am J Geriatr Psychiatry 2009;17(7):542–55.

63. Mukamal KJ. Prospective Study of Alcohol Consumption and Risk of Dementia in Older Adults. JAMA 2003;289(11):1405.

64. Stampfer MJ, Kang JH, Chen J, et al. Effects of moderate alcohol consumption on cognitive function in women. N Engl J Med 2005;352(3):245–53.

65. Bahorik A, Bobrow K, Hoang T, et al. Increased risk of dementia in older female US veterans with alcohol use disorder. Addiction 2021;add:15416.

66. Ownby RL, Crocco E, Acevedo A, et al. Depression and Risk for Alzheimer Disease. Arch Gen Psychiatry 2006;63(5):530.

67. Wilson RS, Barnes LL, Mendes de Leon CF, et al. Depressive symptoms, cognitive decline, and risk of AD in older persons. Neurology 2002;59(3):364–70.

68. Dufouil C, Fuhrer R, Dartigues J-F, et al. Longitudinal analysis of the association between depressive symptomatology and cognitive deterioration. Am J Epidemiol 1996;144(7):634–41.

69. Chen P, Ganguli M, Mulsant BH, et al. The Temporal Relationship Between Depressive Symptoms and Dementia. Arch Gen Psychiatry 1999;56(3):261.

70. Zeki Al Hazzouri A, Vittinghoff E, Byers A, et al. Long-term cumulative depressive symptom burden and risk of cognitive decline and dementia among very old women. Journals Gerontol Ser A Biol Sci Med Sci 2014;69(5):595–601.

71. Heyman A, Wilkinson WE, Stafford JA, et al. Alzheimer's disease: A study of epidemiological aspects. Ann Neurol 1984;15(4):335–41.

72. Kornblith E, Peltz CB, Xia F, et al. Sex, race, and risk of dementia diagnosis after traumatic brain injury among older veterans. Neurology 2020;95(13):e1768–75.

73. Barnes DE, Byers AL, Gardner RC, et al. Association of mild traumatic brain injury with and without loss of consciousness with dementia in US Military Veterans. JAMA Neurol 2018;75(9):1055.

74. Dams-O'Connor K, Gibbons LE, Bowen JD, et al. Risk for late-life re-injury, dementia and death among individuals with traumatic brain injury: a population-based study. J Neurol Neurosurg Psychiatry 2013;84(2):177–82.

75. Lindsay J. Risk Factors for Alzheimer's Disease: A Prospective Analysis from the Canadian Study of Health and Aging. Am J Epidemiol 2002;156(5):445–53.

76. Deschenes CL, McCurry SM. Current treatments for sleep disturbances in individuals with dementia. Curr Psychiatry Rep 2009;11(1):20–6.

77. Leng Y, McEvoy CT, Allen IE, et al. Association of sleep-disordered breathing with cognitive function and risk of cognitive impairment. JAMA Neurol 2017;74(10):1237.

78. Yaffe K, Laffan AM, Harrison SL, et al. Sleep-Disordered Breathing, Hypoxia, and Risk of Mild Cognitive Impairment and Dementia in Older Women. JAMA 2011;306(6). https://doi.org/10.1001/jama.2011.1115.

79. Sexton CE, Sykara K, Karageorgiou E, et al. Connections Between Insomnia and Cognitive Aging. Neurosci Bull 2020;36(1):77–84.

80. Leng Y, Redline S, Stone KL, et al. Objective napping, cognitive decline, and risk of cognitive impairment in older men. Alzheimer's Dement 2019;15(8):1039–47.

81. Chen J, Espeland MA, Brunner RL, et al. Sleep duration, cognitive decline, and dementia risk in older women. Alzheimer's Dement. 2016;12(1):21–33.

82. Ma Y, Liang L, Zheng F, et al. Association Between Sleep Duration and Cognitive Decline. JAMA Netw Open 2020;3(9):e2013573.
83. Blackman J, Swirski M, Clynes J, et al. Pharmacological and non-pharmacological interventions to enhance sleep in mild cognitive impairment and mild Alzheimer's disease: A systematic review. J Sleep Res 2020. https://doi.org/10.1111/jsr.13229.
84. Vellas B, Carrie I, Gillette-Guyonnet S, et al. Mapt Study: a Multidomain Approach for Preventing Alzheimer'S Disease: Design and Baseline Data. J Prev Alzheimer's Dis 2014;1(1):13–22.
85. van Charante EPM, Richard E, Eurelings LS, et al. Effectiveness of a 6-year multidomain vascular care intervention to prevent dementia (preDIVA): a cluster-randomised controlled trial. Lancet 2016;388(10046):797–805.
86. Ngandu T, Lehtisalo J, Solomon A, et al. A 2 year multidomain intervention of diet, exercise, cognitive training, and vascular risk monitoring versus control to prevent cognitive decline in at-risk elderly people (FINGER): a randomised controlled trial. Lancet 2015;385(9984):2255–63.
87. Yaffe K, Barnes DE, Rosenberg D, et al. Systematic Multi-Domain Alzheimer's Risk Reduction Trial (SMARRT): Study Protocol. In: Anstey K, Peters R, editors. J Alzheimer's Dis 2019;70(s1):S207–20.

Psychotic Disorders in the Elderly
Diagnosis, Epidemiology, and Treatment

Corinne E. Fischer, MD[a,b,c,*], Andrew Namasivayam, MD[b,1],
Lucas Crawford-Holland, BA & Sc Cand[a], Narek Hakobyan, BSc[a],
Tom A. Schweizer, PhD[a,c,d], David G. Munoz, MD, MSc[a,c,e],
Bruce G. Pollock, MD, PhD[f,g]

KEYWORDS

- Elderly • Schizophrenia • Schizoaffective disorder • Delusional disorder • Psychosis
- Citalopram • Pimavanserin • Alzheimer disease

KEY POINTS

- Psychotic symptoms are prevalent in older patients referred for psychiatric evaluation.
- Clinical challenges emerge due to the variety of diagnostic possibilities in older patients with no prior psychosis history.
- Age of onset and clinical features distinguish patients with early versus late-onset psychotic disorders.
- Revised research and clinical criteria for dementia-related psychosis emphasize the occurrence of symptoms across the neurodegenerative spectrum.
- New therapies for dementia-related psychosis such as citalopram and pimavanserin offer new treatment options.

INTRODUCTION

Psychotic symptoms are a frequent occurrence among older patients referred for psychiatric evaluation. In patients with existing diagnoses including bipolar disorder,

[a] Keenan Research Centre for Biomedical Science, Room 17044 cc wing, St. Michaels Hospital, #30 Bond St., Toronto, Ontario, M5B1W8, Canada; [b] Department of Psychiatry, University of Toronto, Toronto, Ontario, Canada; [c] St. Michael's Hospital, 30 Bond Street, Toronto, Ontario M5B 1W8, Canada; [d] Department of Neurosurgery, University of Toronto, Toronto, Canada; [e] Department of Laboratory Medicine and Pathobiology, University of Toronto, Toronto, Canada; [f] Division of Geriatric Psychiatry, Campbell Family Mental Health Research Institute, Centre for Addiction and Mental Health, 250 College Street, Toronto, Ontario, M5T 1R8, Canada; [g] Toronto Dementia Research Alliance, University of Toronto, Toronto, Ontario, Canada
[1] Present address: 30 Bond St. Toronto, Ontario M5B 1W8, Canada.
* Corresponding author. St. Michael's Hospital, 30 Bond Street, Toronto, Ontario M5B 1W8, Canada.
E-mail address: corinne.fischer@unityhealth.to

Psychiatr Clin N Am 45 (2022) 691–705
https://doi.org/10.1016/j.psc.2022.07.001
0193-953X/22/© 2022 Elsevier Inc. All rights reserved.
psych.theclinics.com

schizophrenia, and psychotic depression, the diagnosis and associated treatments may be quite straightforward. However, the de novo presentation of psychotic symptoms in older persons with no prior history presents several clinical challenges. Could the symptoms be the first manifestation of an emerging neurocognitive disorder? Could they represent a late-life psychiatric disorder such as late-life delusional disorder or late-life schizophrenia? Alternatively, could they be provoked by accumulating sensory deficits as in Charles Bonnet syndrome? The list of diagnostic possibilities and the absence of specific disease-related biomarkers make this all the more challenging. In the last 5 years, there have been important new developments in our characterization of psychosis in the context of neurocognitive disorders. It is being increasingly recognized with constructs such as mild behavioral impairment (MBI) that neuropsychiatric symptoms (NPS), including psychosis, might be a *forme fruste* of dementia. Additionally, the emergence of novel infections such as severe acute respiratory syndrome coronavirus 2 and anti-N-methyl-D-aspartate (NMDA) encephalitis has broadened our understanding of the important link between disease, inflammation, and psychosis. Moreover, new therapies such as citalopram and pimavanserin for dementia-related psychosis offer new treatment options. In the following review, we will discuss the latest advances in diagnosis, epidemiology, and treatment as it pertains to psychosis in the elderly.

Diagnosis

Early-onset schizophrenia

A proportion of older patients with psychotic symptoms will be diagnosed with schizophrenia. Most of these patients will already have an established diagnosis of schizophrenia diagnosed at a much younger age although a minority of patients may develop symptoms for the first time later in life. DSM-V and ICD-10 criteria outline what symptoms constitute a diagnosis.[1] These include at least 2 of 5 core symptoms, delusions, hallucinations, disorganized speech, disorganized or catatonic behavior, and negative symptoms. Patients who develop symptoms of schizophrenia at a typical age of onset, in their 20s or 30s, will age and longitudinal studies do suggest an improved treatment trajectory for those that survive.[2] A World Health Organization study followed patients with schizophrenia prospectively for 15 to 25 years and cited favorable outcomes in approximately 50% of patients.[2] An important caveat to this finding is that milder symptoms of schizophrenia favor survival to an older age.

Late-onset/very late-onset schizophrenia

Of patients with schizophrenia, it is estimated that approximately 25% of cases will be diagnosed later in life, on or after the age of 40.[3] Debate continues as to what extent patients with late-onset schizophrenia (LOS) differ from patients with early-onset schizophrenia (EOS), although clinical differences have been observed. An international consensus conference in 2000 concluded that the first onset of symptoms between 40 and 60 years should constitute LOS and the onset of symptoms after age 60 should constitute very late-onset schizophrenia (VLOS).[4] Studies suggest certain overlapping features between EOS and LOS, including minor physical anomalies[5] and sensory deficits.[6] Differentiating factors in LOS include greater preponderance in women,[7] lower rates of family history,[8] and preserved psychosocial functioning among other features.[3,9]

Delusional disorder/schizoaffective disorder

The existing literature in older patients with other psychotic disorders such as delusional disorder and schizoaffective disorder is quite limited. Comparable to the data on schizophrenia, the onset of symptoms after age 40 demarcates patients with late-onset delusional disorder, whereas onset after age 60 demarcates patients with very late-onset delusional disorder. Schizoaffective disorder, according to DSM-V, does require the presence of sustained delusions/hallucinations as well as a major mood component that may occur concurrently with the psychotic symptoms. Studies on late-onset/very late-onset schizoaffective disorder remain scant although the conventional cutoff age of 40 years for late-onset and 60 years for very late-onset may apply following consensus guidelines.[4]

Affective disorders

Most patients with psychotic depression develop mood-congruent delusions, which tend to be nihilistic. These include guilt, poverty, punishment, somatic delusions, and feelings of inadequacy.[10] Auditory voice hallucinations may occur in some instances.[10] Patients with bipolar disorder, whether early or late in onset, may manifest psychotic symptoms. Typical symptoms include grandiose beliefs if manic or nihilistic delusions if depressed.

Isolated psychotic symptoms

Isolated psychotic symptoms, specifically spontaneous visual or auditory hallucinations in the absence of other symptoms, may occur with the aging process. These symptoms may consist of benign images or sounds such as music, and so forth. These isolated symptoms are thought to be more common than disorders, are typically associated with preserved insight, and do not cause significant stress.[11]

Psychosis and cognitive impairment

Psychotic symptoms in older adults may be an early signal of an oncoming neurodegenerative disorder.[12,13] The newly revised clinical criteria[14] and research framework[15] for dementia-related psychosis do suggest a shift in thinking, with the clinical criteria allowing for the emergence of symptoms in the mild cognitive impairment (MCI) phase and the research framework allowing for diagnosis of symptoms in the preclinical phase if biomarkers are confirmatory of neurodegeneration (**Table 1**).

Psychotic symptoms in Alzheimer disease

Psychotic symptoms have been studied most extensively in Alzheimer disease (AD), where they consist of delusions and hallucinations under newly established criteria.[14,15] Delusions generally are divided into persecutory and misidentification delusions,[16] with the latter occurring later in the disease course and thought to indicate more misremembering reflective of hippocampal damage.[17] Visual hallucinations may occur in patients with AD and advanced cognitive decline and have not been well-characterized. Significant overlap between delusions and hallucinations may occur not uncommonly although symptoms may be separate in 10% to 20% of cases.[18]

Psychotic symptoms in Lewy body dementia and Parkinson disease dementia

Other forms of neurodegeneration such as alpha synucleinopathies may be associated with a higher frequency of psychotic symptoms, in particular vivid visual hallucinations consisting of shadows, animals, and so forth. Dementia with Lewy bodies (DLB) is associated with a high prevalence of such symptoms and constitutes a core diagnostic criterion, along with fluctuations and parkinsonism.[19] Parkinson's disease dementia (PDD) has an equally high prevalence of such symptoms, which range from minor to complex hallucinations.[20,21] Minor hallucinations typically consist of illusions, where a stimulus is misperceived as something else. One common type is referred to as "pareidolia," where meaningful images are formed from random visual scenes. "Passage" (consisting of shadows observed out of the corner of one's eye)

Table 1
Comparison of research-based and clinical criteria for dementia-related psychosis

Criteria	ISTAART Dementia-related psychosis framework	Psychosis in Major and Mild Neurocognitive Disorder: International Psychogeriatric Association (IPA) Consensus Clinical and Research Definition
Diagnosis	National Institute of Aging Criteria Focus on the AD spectrum but symptoms may be preclinical	DSM-V criteria Symptoms must be in the MCI range and occur across the neurogenerative spectrum
Duration	1 mo	1 mo
Symptoms	Delusions and hallucinations but note made of subtypes of symptoms and persistent/ fluctuating	Delusions and hallucinations included, examples provided of each
Exclusions	Delirium, primary psychotic illness, a general medical condition or an agitation/affective syndrome	Delirium, primary psychotic illness, a general medical condition. Affective and agitation syndromes are noted but are not exclusions
Severity and chronology	No reference to function. Symptoms may precede cognitive decline	Symptoms must affect function beyond that of the underlying dementia. Symptoms must follow cognitive impairment not precede it

and "presence" (consisting of the belief that someone is standing next to the patient) hallucinations may also occur, as well as delusions although they tend to be rare.

Psychotic symptoms in frontal temporal dementia

Psychotic symptoms are being observed with increasing frequency in patients with frontal temporal dementia (FTD), in particular among those with chromosome 9 open reading frame 72 repeats who test positive for transactive response DNA-binding protein 43.[22] Delusions, somatic obsessions, and multimodal hallucinations tend to predominate.[22]

Psychotic symptoms in general medical conditions

Psychotic symptoms may occur in the context of many neurologic, infectious, neoplastic, and inflammatory conditions. Autoimmune encephalitis is an important consideration given the recent availability of autoantibody panels. Psychotic symptoms have not been well-characterized, although they are frequently seen in association with other neuropsychiatric features.[23] Coronavirus disease (COVID-19) infection may cause psychotic symptoms in older adults but further studies are required to more carefully delineate the symptom presentation.[24]

Clinics Care Points

- Late-life psychiatric presentation including schizophrenia, schizoaffective disorder, and delusional disorder are defined by the age of-onset with after 40 years constituting late onset and after 60 years constituting very late-onset.
- Certain features distinguish early from late-onset presentations.
- Psychotic symptoms may, in some cases, be a presenting manifestation of dementia and certain phenomenological characteristics make this more likely.

Epidemiology

Nonaffective psychosis and schizophrenia

Schizophrenia is a psychotic disorder that can also be divided into the 3 stages of onset mentioned previously: early-onset, late-onset, which has a lifetime prevalence of 1%, and very late-onset with a lifetime prevalence of 0.3%[25] in the general population. LOS has been shown to have a higher frequency in diagnosis overall, and women are more frequently diagnosed than men (**Table 2**).[26]

Affective psychosis

Psychotic depression has a lifetime prevalence of 0.35% and psychosis has a 20% to 45% prevalence in patients hospitalized with depression.[25] Psychotic depression can be categorized into similar stages of onset to schizophrenia with an average age of onset being 51 years. Patients with late-onset have more severe depression but less frequent paranoia and have similar rates of psychosis, compared with early-onset psychotic depression.[25] It is estimated that 0.25% to 1% of the elderly have bipolar disorder, for whom late-onset mania has a 44% prevalence (see **Table 2**).[27]

Delusional disorder

Determining the exact prevalence is difficult due to historically inconsistent and vague diagnostic criteria; however, it has been estimated as having a lifetime prevalence of 0.18%.[25] Delusional disorder typically affects older adults with a mean onset age of 48.76 years (see **Table 2**).[25]

Dementia-related psychosis

The most common cause of late-life psychosis is dementia. AD, vascular dementia, Parkinson's disease (PD), and DLB can result in dementia-related psychosis. In

Table 2	
Prevalence of psychosis in various disorders and diseases	
Disorder Type	**Prevalence of Psychosis**
Primary Psychoses	
Schizophrenia	Lifetime prevalence • 1% late-onset • 0.3% very late-onset
Depression	Lifetime prevalence: 0.35%
Bipolar disorder	Prevalence in elderly population: 0.25%–1%
Delusional disorder	Lifetime prevalence: 0.18%
Mild behavioral impairment	3% in cognitively normal MBI patients
Dementia (all types)	20%–70%
Alzheimer disease	30%–50%
Parkinson disease	40% • More than 50% in those with PD dementia
DLB	75%
Vascular dementia	15%
FTD	10%
Secondary Psychoses	
Substance use	Accounts for 10% of all causes of late-life psychosis
Delirium	>40%
COVID-19	0.9%–4%

dementia, psychosis has a prevalence of 20% to 70%[28] and increases with disease progression and greater cognitive decline (see **Table 2**).[28]

Alzheimer disease
In AD dementia, psychotic symptoms are present in 30% to 50% of cases.[15,25] Hallucinations and delusions are found in around 10% to 20% and 15% to 40% of AD cases, respectively.[25,28] Dementia severity has also been positively correlated with psychosis presence and severity (see **Table 2**).[25]

Parkinson disease
Determining the exact prevalence of psychosis in PD is difficult because antiparkinsonian drugs may themselves cause psychotic symptoms. However, the prevalence of psychosis in PD is reported as around 40%.[25,29] More than 30% of patients with PD have dementia, and dementia is a significant risk factor for developing psychosis in PD. As such, the prevalence of psychosis in PD patients with dementia has been reported as at least 50%.[28] The presence of visual hallucinations and dementia are positively correlated in PD. However, psychosis severity and dementia severity tend not to be associated with each other (see **Table 2**).[25]

Dementia with Lewy Bodies
Another disease that commonly exhibits dementia psychosis is DLB. Psychosis is very common in DLB, with prevalence reported as high as 75%.[28] Unlike PD, dementia severity and psychosis severity seem to be positively correlated in DLB (see **Table 2**).[25]

Other sources of dementia
Psychosis in vascular dementia and frontotemporal dementia are less common than in other cases of dementia. In vascular dementia, psychosis has been found in around 15% of patients, with delusions more common than hallucinations.[14] The severity of dementia is associated with neither psychotic symptom prevalence nor severity. FTD has the lowest prevalence of psychosis at 10%, with delusions being the most common psychotic symptom (see **Table 2**).[14]

Mild Behavioral Impairment
MBI serves as a diagnostic framework to assess NPS in later life and helps to determine risk levels for all-cause dementia. One of the 5 domains of MBI is the presence of psychotic symptoms. The prevalence of psychosis has been found as low as 3% in cognitively normal MBI patients (see **Table 2**).[30]

Secondary psychosis
Psychoses are deemed secondary when substance use or underlying medical disorders are causing psychotic symptoms. Secondary psychosis may be categorized into substance/medication-induced psychotic disorder, delirium, and disease. Psychosis caused by substance use and withdrawal accounts for 10% of all causes of late-life psychosis. Delirium is another source of secondary psychosis, characterized by rapid and dramatic fluctuations in awareness and attention. Twenty-three percent of hospitalized older adults are diagnosed with delirium. Delirium is estimated as responsible for 10% of late-life psychoses,[27] with more than 40% of delirium patients exhibiting psychotic symptoms (see **Table 2**).[31]

Coronavirus infection
Evidence has emerged that COVID-19 increases the risk of psychosis, with estimates that 0.9% to 4% of those infected with Sars-CoV-2 develop psychosis.[31] COVID-19 infection

severity may increase this risk. However, it is unclear whether the risk varies with age (see **Table 2**).

CLINICS CARE PEARLS

- Life-time prevalence of late-life psychotic disorders range in prevalence from 0.3% to 1%.
- Prevalence in dementia increases with severity and is higher in certain subtypes of dementia (DLB, PDD).
- Sars-CoV-2 may be a rare cause of psychosis in older patients (see **Table 2**).

Treatment

Late-onset schizophrenia and very late-onset schizophrenia-like psychosis

Two Cochrane reviews from 2003 and 2012 concluded that there was no trial-based evidence on which to base guidelines for antipsychotic use in LOS.[32,33] Older retrospective studies on antipsychotic effectiveness in LOS and VLOS-like psychosis (VLOSLP) showed that 48% to 61% of patients had complete remission of symptoms.[4] In 2018, Howard and colleagues published the first randomized-controlled trial (RCT) assessing antipsychotic efficacy in VLOSLP.[34] The study demonstrated that amisulpride 100 mg/d produced significant improvement in the Brief Psychiatric Rating Scale compared with placebo during 12 weeks of treatment. In a small open-label study, amisulpride 50 mg/d was also found to produce a clinically relevant response.[35]

Currently, the dosing of antipsychotics in patients with late-life primary psychosis is largely based on consensus derived from a 2004 survey of 48 experts in geriatric psychiatry and geriatric medicine.[36] The consensus article recommends using lower doses than those typically used in younger patients: the first-choice recommendation is risperidone 1.25 to 3.5 mg/d, and the second-choice recommendations are quetiapine 100 to 300 mg/d, olanzapine 7.5 to 15 mg/d, or aripiprazole 15 to 30 mg/d (**Table 3**).

The recommendation for lower antipsychotic doses reflects the notion that sensitivity to both the therapeutic and adverse effects of antipsychotics increases with age.[37] This is due to age-related pharmacokinetic and pharmacodynamic changes, as well as higher rates of comorbidity and polypharmacy in the elderly. Compared with typical antipsychotics, atypical antipsychotics are less likely to produce parkinsonism and tardive dyskinesia[37] but studies have not demonstrated a significant difference in falls risk between the 2 classes.[38] Although there is mounting evidence to support the use of lower antipsychotic dosages in the elderly, in general, there is very limited data on dosing for late-onset and very late-onset primary psychotic disorders specifically.

Psychosocial treatments

RCTs have demonstrated the effectiveness of various psychosocial treatments for improving function in older patients with schizophrenia.[39] Such treatments include functional adaptation skills training, cognitive-behavioral social skills training, supported employment, and other intensive skills training programs.

Delusional disorder

Treatment of late-life delusional disorder is guided by the evidence base established in younger patients, and there is a need for additional research on this topic. A recent descriptive study examined long-term treatment outcomes of 55 geriatric patients with delusional disorder of mostly persecutory type.[40] In patients treated with atypical antipsychotics, most of whom were hospitalized, 35% showed clinical improvement and 20% had sustained absence of discernible symptoms after an average of

Table 3
Summary of treatments for psychosis in the elderly

Delirium or Medical Illness	Treat Primary Medical Problem	N/A
Depression	Antidepressant plus atypical antipsychotic	Expert consensus (RCTs support olanzapine plus sertraline)[42–44]
	ECT	Expert consensus[44]
Bipolar disorder	Atypical antipsychotic (olanzapine, risperidone, quetiapine, and clozapine)	Ranges from case studies to secondary analyses of RCTs[45]
	Lithium or divalproex monotherapy may be sufficient	RCT[46]
Delusional disorder	Atypical antipsychotic (especially oral and intramuscular risperidone, and intramuscular paliperidone)	Retrospective study[40]
VLOSLP	Risperidone 1.25–3.5 mg/d, quetiapine 100–300 mg/d, olanzapine 7.5–15 mg/d, or aripiprazole 15–30 mg/d	Expert consensus[36]
	Amisulpride 100 mg/d	RCTs[34]
AD	Citalopram 20–30 mg/d	RCTs[47–49]
	Atypical antipsychotics (particularly risperidone and aripiprazole), some data emerging for pimavanserin, note increased mortality risk	RCTs and meta-analyses[54]
Frontotemporal dementia	Atypical antipsychotics	Case reports/series[59,60]
	ECT	
Parkinson disease	Rivastigmine or donepezil	Case series to RCTs[62]
	Pimavanserin or clozapine	RCTs[63]
	Quetiapine, aripiprazole, risperidone, and ziprasidone have mixed evidence	Expert opinion, case studies open trials[62,63]
DLB	Donepezil	Various studies including RCTs[65]
	Low-dose olanzapine, aripiprazole, quetiapine, and clozapine	Mostly case reports/series[65]

Abbreviations: ECT, electroconvulsive therapy; RCT, randomized control trial; VLOSLP, very late-onset schizophrenia-like psychosis

36 months of follow-up. The antipsychotics most commonly used were oral risperidone, intramuscular risperidone, and intramuscular paliperidone palmitate. Resolution of symptoms was typically achieved after 2 to 8 months of antipsychotic treatment (see **Table 3**).

Psychotic depression

There is a shortage of studies on the treatment of psychotic depression specifically in the elderly. Small studies of antidepressant monotherapy in this population have found treatment response rates ranging from 18% to 44%.[41] Two small RCTs found that the combination of nortriptyline and perphenazine was not significantly more efficacious than nortriptyline alone in either the acute (mean 9 weeks) or maintenance (6 months) treatment phases.[41] However, in the larger study of pharmacotherapy of psychotic depression (STOP-PD) trial, treatment during 12 weeks with olanzapine plus sertraline was superior to olanzapine plus placebo in older patients.[42] In the STOP-PD II trial, patients who received olanzapine plus sertraline were less likely to relapse during 36 weeks compared with those who received sertraline plus placebo, although the former group experienced more weight gain.[43] These recent trials support the recommendation from existing guidelines of treating late-life psychotic depression with an antidepressant plus an atypical antipsychotic.[44] Furthermore, electroconvulsive therapy (ECT) is indicated for psychotic depression in the elderly and has evidence to support this, although from a limited number of studies (see **Table 3**).41

Psychosis in bipolar disorder

In clinical practice, psychosis as part of acute mania is often treated with antipsychotics, sometimes in combination with a mood stabilizer. Published evidence in the geriatric population, although sparse, demonstrates the effectiveness of olanzapine, risperidone, quetiapine, and clozapine.[45] In the recent GERI-BD trial, although 34% of participants had mania with psychosis initially, after treatment with either lithium or divalproex, less than 20% of participants required an adjunctive antipsychotic.[46] This suggests that more frequent use of lithium or divalproex may obviate an antipsychotic (see **Table 3**).

Alzheimer disease

Antidepressants. Citalopram has demonstrated efficacy for agitation and psychosis in patients with AD in RCTs. Separate trials showed that it was superior to perphenazine and placebo[47] and equivalent to risperidone while producing fewer side effects.[48] The CitAD trial demonstrated that in patients with AD, citalopram 30 mg/d was superior to placebo in reducing agitation.[49] A secondary analysis found that citalopram-treated individuals also had a reduction in delusions and hallucinations.[50] However, concerns about QTc prolongation and worsening cognition at this dose of citalopram limit its clinical utility.[49] Escitalopram, which is relatively safer, is currently being investigated as a treatment of agitation in AD in the S-CitAD trial, and psychosis will be a secondary outcome measure (see **Table 3**).[51]

Antipsychotics. In the treatment of psychosis in AD, studies have shown that antipsychotics confer modest benefits while carrying a risk of considerable adverse effects, including mortality. The clinical antipsychotic trials of intervention effectiveness (CATIE)-AD trial investigated the effectiveness of atypical antipsychotics for psychosis and agitation in 421 AD patients.[52] After 36 weeks of treatment, no significant differences were noted among treatment groups (risperidone, olanzapine, quetiapine, placebo) with respect to the primary treatment outcome, time to discontinuation of treatment for any reason. Olanzapine and risperidone were favored based on the primary efficacy measure, time to discontinuation. In a last observation carried forward analysis using the data from the 12-week time point of the trial, olanzapine and risperidone were shown to be effective for reducing hostility and paranoid delusions.[53] However, meta-analyses of datasets from multiple trials have shown that risperidone and aripiprazole have the most evidence for efficacy, with the latter likely being the safest option as well (see **Table 3**).[54]

More recently, pimavanserin has emerged as an effective antipsychotic for treatment of psychosis in dementia. In 2021, results were published from a phase 3 trial consisting of an open-label phase followed by a double-blind phase.[55] Of the 351 patients who received open-label pimavanserin for 12 weeks, 217 had a positive response at the 8-week and 12-week time points, and these patients were then randomized to either continue receiving pimavanserin or switched to placebo. Patients in the pimavanserin group were significantly less likely to experience a relapse of psychosis, necessitating early stoppage of the trial (see **Table 3**).

The substantial adverse effects associated with antipsychotic use in this population require clinicians to exercise prudence when deciding whether to prescribe. In 2005, the US Food and Drug Administration issued a warning that the use of atypical antipsychotics to treat behavioral disturbances in elderly patients with dementia increased the risk of death by 1.6 to 1.7 times.[56] In meta-analyses, risperidone and olanzapine have been associated with an increased risk of cerebrovascular adverse events relative to placebo.[54]

Lithium. The LitAD trial was a 12-week study investigating the effects of lithium on agitation in 77 patients with AD.[57] The trial showed that lithium 150 to 600 mg/d was not superior to placebo in reducing agitation but was superior in improving clinical global impression and reducing delusions, whereas not worsening cognition. Further research is needed to clarify the role of lithium in AD psychosis (see **Table 3**).

Frontotemporal dementia. There have been no systematic studies specifically for the treatment of psychosis in FTD. In practice, medications used for psychosis related to AD and psychiatric disorders are used off-label in FTD.[58] From the handful of case studies that have been published, some have reported improvement of psychosis with atypical antipsychotics or ECT, whereas others have reported symptom persistence despite antipsychotic treatment.[59,60] Importantly, patients with FTD may be at increased risk of developing extrapyramidal symptoms from antipsychotic use,[59] and therefore these medications should be administered judiciously. Preference is sometimes given to antipsychotics with low D2 receptor occupancy (eg, quetiapine).

Parkinson's disease dementia

In patients with Parkinson's disease, psychotic symptoms often resolve once secondary causes, such as systemic illnesses or dopaminergic medications, are addressed.[61] If symptoms persist, an acetylcholinesterase inhibitor should be considered first.[62] There is modest evidence for both donepezil and rivastigmine in the treatment of visual hallucinations in Parkinson disease, with more consistent efficacy reported for rivastigmine.[62] The NMDA antagonist memantine is not recommended for treating psychosis in this population because it has been shown to worsen psychotic symptoms.[62]

Antipsychotics should be reserved for those patients in whom other treatments have failed and psychotic symptoms are impairing function, causing distress, or posing a safety concern.[62] Typical antipsychotics should be avoided because they can worsen motor symptoms via dopaminergic blockade. Of the atypical antipsychotics, the 2 that are supported by double-blind placebo-controlled trials are clozapine and pimavanserin, although longer term data are lacking for both.[63]

Compared with clozapine and pimavanserin, other atypical antipsychotics do not have as strong of an evidence base to support their use for this indication. Quetiapine was shown to be efficacious in open-label studies but not in 3 RCTs.[63] However, quetiapine was shown to not worsen motor function, and many clinicians use it in low doses (25–75 mg/d) as a first-line treatment based on clinical experience and expert opinion.[63] Risperidone, aripiprazole, and ziprasidone have mixed results from open-label studies and case series.[62] Olanzapine has been shown in clinical trials to worsen motor function while conferring no benefit for psychosis (see **Table 3**).[63]

For Parkinson's disease patients with psychosis and comorbid depression or anxiety, there have been some case reports of antidepressant monotherapy or adjunct therapy reducing psychotic symptoms.[64]

Dementia with Lewy Bodies

High-quality evidence to guide the treatment of psychosis in DLB is lacking. Donepezil 5 to 10 mg/d has some evidence for treating psychotic symptoms, particularly hallucinations, whereas rivastigmine, galantamine, and memantine do not.[65] Patients with DLB can have an exquisite, and sometimes fatal, sensitivity to antipsychotics, with potential reactions including autonomic dysfunction, impaired consciousness, and a worsening of their parkinsonism.[66] Therefore, antipsychotics, especially typical antipsychotics, should be avoided in this population if possible. A recent meta-analysis proposed that based on the available evidence, low-dose olanzapine, aripiprazole, quetiapine, and clozapine can be considered if necessary, with olanzapine having the best evidence, although it may worsen motor symptoms.[65] In practice, quetiapine or aripiprazole is often used because they are thought to be better tolerated and have less effect on motor symptoms (see **Table 3**).

CLINICS CARE POINTS

- Expert consensus and RCT data favors atypical antipsychotics in late-life psychotic disorders.
- Citalopram, escitalopram, and pimavanserin based on RCT data have shown promising effects in older patients with dementia-related psychosis.
- Low-dose atypical antipsychotics based on RCT data may be useful in dementia-related psychosis but consideration should be given to increased mortality risk.

SUMMARY

Late-life psychotic disorders continue to be defined by age of onset with late onset symptoms emerging after age 40 and very late-onset emerging after age 60. New research and clinical criteria for dementia-related psychosis will likely affect the prevalence rates of psychosis in dementia, which presently only include symptoms that emerge after a diagnosis of dementia. The presence of psychosis in a patient with minimal cognitive symptoms and biomarkers suggestive of dementia would have previously been classified as late-life psychosis but now might be recategorized as dementia-related psychosis. This will likely have implications for the treatment as well, given the presence of neurodegeneration increases mortality associated with the use of antipsychotic medication. Expert consensus and RCT data continue to support the use of atypical antipsychotic medications in patients with late-life psychosis, although caution is necessary when using such treatments in dementia-related psychosis due to increased mortality risk. Citalopram and pimavanserin are promising treatments based on recent RCT data. Future mechanistically based studies as well as new insights learned from the study of emerging pathogens including SAR-Cov2 will further inform our understanding of psychosis in the elderly.

Dr B.G. Pollock's research study is supported in part by the Peter & Shelagh Godsoe Endowed Chair in Late-Life Mental Health

ACKNOWLEDGMENTS

Dr. Pollock's research work is supported in part by the Peter & Shelagh Godsoe Endowed Chair in Late-Life Mental Health

DISCLOSURE

Dr B.G. Pollock holds United States Provisional Patent Nos. 6/490,680, 17/396,030 and Canadian Provisional Patent No. 3,054,093 for a cell-based assay and kits for assessing serum anticholinergic activity. Dr C.E. Fischer receives grant funding from Hoffman La Roche and Vielight Inc.

REFERENCES

1. American Psychiatric Association. American Psychiatric Association. DSM-5 Task Force. Diagnostic and statistical manual of mental disorders: DSM-5. 5th edition. Arlington, VA: American Psychiatric Association; 2013. p. xliv, 947.
2. Harrison G, Hopper K, Craig T, et al. Recovery from psychotic illness: a 15- and 25-year international follow-up study. Br J Psychiatry 2001;178:506–17.
3. Harris MJ, Jeste DV. Late-onset schizophrenia: an overview. Schizophr Bull 1988; 14(1):39–55.
4. Howard R, Rabins PV, Seeman MV, et al. Late-onset schizophrenia and very-late-onset schizophrenia-like psychosis: an international consensus. the international late-onset schizophrenia group. Am J Psychiatry 2000;157(2):172–8.
5. Lohr JB, Alder M, Flynn K, et al. Minor physical anomalies in older patients with late-onset schizophrenia, early-onset schizophrenia, depression, and Alzheimer's disease. *Am J Geriatr Psychiatry* Fall 1997;5(4):318–23.
6. Jeste DV, Symonds LL, Harris MJ, et al. Nondementia Nonpraecox Dementia Praecox?: Late-Onset Schizophrenia. Am J Geriatr Psychiatry 1997;5(4):302–17.
7. Castle DJ, Murray RM. The epidemiology of late-onset schizophrenia. Schizophr Bull 1993;19(4):691–700.
8. Howard RJ, Graham C, Sham P, et al. A controlled family study of late-onset non-affective psychosis (late paraphrenia). Br J Psychiatry 1997;170:511–4.
9. Alici-Evcimen Y, Ertan T, Eker E. Case series with late-onset psychosis hospitalized in a geriatric psychiatry unit in Turkey: experience in 9 years. Int Psychogeriatr 2003;15(1):69–72.
10. Meyers BS, Klimstra SA, Gabriele M, et al. Continuation treatment of delusional depression in older adults. *Am J Geriatr Psychiatry* Fall 2001;9(4):415–22.
11. Shoham N, Lewis G, Hayes J, et al. Psychotic symptoms and sensory impairment: Findings from the 2014 adult psychiatric morbidity survey. Schizophr Res 2020;215:357–64.
12. Peters ME, Schwartz S, Han D, et al. Neuropsychiatric symptoms as predictors of progression to severe Alzheimer's dementia and death: the Cache County Dementia Progression Study. Am J Psychiatry 2015;172(5):460–5.
13. Fischer CE, Agüera-Ortiz L. Psychosis and dementia: risk factor, prodrome, or cause? Int Psychogeriatr 2018;30(2):209–19.
14. Cummings J, Pinto LC, Cruz M, et al. Criteria for psychosis in major and mild neurocognitive disorders: international psychogeriatric association (ipa) consensus clinical and research definition. Am J Geriatr Psychiatry 2020;28(12):1256–69.
15. Fischer CE, Ismail Z, Youakim JM, et al. Revisiting criteria for psychosis in alzheimer's disease and related dementias: toward better phenotypic classification and biomarker research. J Alzheimers Dis 2020;73(3):1143–56.
16. Cook SE, Miyahara S, Bacanu S-A, et al. Psychotic symptoms in alzheimer disease: evidence for subtypes. Am J Geriatr Psychiatry 2003;11(4):406–13.
17. Perez-Madrinan G, Cook SE, Saxton JA, et al. Alzheimer disease with psychosis: excess cognitive impairment is restricted to the misidentification subtype. Am J Geriatr Psychiatry 2004;12(5):449–56.

18. Connors MH, Ames D, Woodward M, et al. Psychosis and clinical outcomes in alzheimer disease: a longitudinal study. Am J Geriatr Psychiatry 2018;26(3): 304–13.
19. Yamada M, Komatsu J, Nakamura K, et al. Diagnostic criteria for dementia with lewy bodies: updates and future directions. J Mov Disord 2020;13(1):1–10.
20. Lenka A, Pagonabarraga J, Pal PK, et al. Minor hallucinations in Parkinson disease: A subtle symptom with major clinical implications. Neurology 2019;93(6): 259–66.
21. Lenka A, Kamat A, Mittal SO. Spectrum of movement disorders in patients with neuroinvasive west nile virus infection. Mov Disord Clin Pract 2019;6(6):426–33.
22. Naasan G, Shdo SM, Rodriguez EM, et al. Psychosis in neurodegenerative disease: differential patterns of hallucination and delusion symptoms. Brain 2021; 144(3):999–1012.
23. Finke C. A transdiagnostic pattern of psychiatric symptoms in autoimmune encephalitis. Lancet Psychiatry 2019;6(3):191–3.
24. Desai S, Sheikh B, Belzie L. New-onset psychosis following COVID-19 infection. Cureus 2021;13(9):e17904.
25. Colijn MA, Nitta BH, Grossberg GT. Psychosis in later life: a review and update. Harv Rev Psychiatry 2015;23(5):354–67.
26. Stafford J, Howard R, Kirkbride JB. The incidence of very late-onset psychotic disorders: a systematic review and meta-analysis, 1960-2016. Psychol Med 2018;48(11):1775–86.
27. Reinhardt MM, Cohen CI. Late-life psychosis: diagnosis and treatment. Curr Psychiatry Rep 2015;17(2):1.
28. Cummings J, Ballard C, Tariot P, et al. Pimavanserin: potential treatment for dementia-related psychosis. J Prev Alzheimers Dis 2018;5(4):253–8.
29. Fénelon G, Mahieux F, Huon R, et al. Hallucinations in Parkinson's disease: prevalence, phenomenology and risk factors. Brain 2000;123(Pt 4):733–45.
30. Ruthirakuhan M, Ismail Z, Herrmann N, et al. Mild behavioral impairment is associated with progression to Alzheimer's disease: A clinicopathological study. Alzheimers Dement 2022. https://doi.org/10.1002/alz.12519. Online ahead of print.
31. Dinakaran D, Manjunatha N, Naveen Kumar C, et al. Neuropsychiatric aspects of COVID-19 pandemic: a selective review. Asian J Psychiatr 2020;53:102188.
32. Arunpongpaisal S, Ahmed I, Aqeel N, et al. Antipsychotic drug treatment for elderly people with late-onset schizophrenia. Cochrane Database Syst Rev 2003;2:CD004162.
33. Essali A, Ali G. Antipsychotic drug treatment for elderly people with late-onset schizophrenia. Cochrane Database Syst Rev 2012;2:CD004162.
34. Howard R, Cort E, Bradley R, et al. Antipsychotic treatment of very late-onset schizophrenia-like psychosis (ATLAS): a randomised, controlled, double-blind trial. Lancet Psychiatry 2018;5(7):553–63.
35. Reeves S, Eggleston K, Cort E, et al. Therapeutic D2/3 receptor occupancies and response with low amisulpride blood concentrations in very late-onset schizophrenia-like psychosis (VLOSLP). Int J Geriatr Psychiatry 2018;33(2):396–404.
36. Alexopoulos GS, Streim J, Carpenter D, et al. Expert consensus panel for using antipsychotic drugs in older p. using antipsychotic agents in older patients. J Clin Psychiatry 2004;65(Suppl 2):5–99 ; discussion 100-102; quiz 103-4.
37. Leon C, Gerretsen P, Uchida H, et al. Sensitivity to antipsychotic drugs in older adults. Curr Psychiatry Rep 2010;12(1):28–33.
38. Huang AR, Mallet L, Rochefort CM, et al. Medication-related falls in the elderly: causative factors and preventive strategies. Drugs Aging 2012;29(5):359–76.

39. Jeste DV, Maglione JE. Treating older adults with schizophrenia: challenges and opportunities. Schizophr Bull 2013;39(5):966–98.
40. Nagendra J, Snowdon J. An Australian study of delusional disorder in late life. Int Psychogeriatr 2020;32(4):453–62.
41. Gournellis R, Oulis P, Howard R. Psychotic major depression in older people: a systematic review. Int J Geriatr Psychiatry 2014;29(8):789–96.
42. Meyers BS, Flint AJ, Rothschild AJ, et al. A double-blind randomized controlled trial of olanzapine plus sertraline vs olanzapine plus placebo for psychotic depression: the study of pharmacotherapy of psychotic depression (STOP-PD). Arch Gen Psychiatry 2009;66(8):838–47.
43. Flint AJ, Meyers BS, Rothschild AJ, et al. Effect of continuing olanzapine vs placebo on relapse among patients with psychotic depression in remission: the stop-pd ii randomized clinical trial. JAMA 2019;322(7):622–31.
44. Alexopoulos GS, Katz IR, Reynolds CF 3rd, et al. Expert consensus panel for pharmacotherapy of depressive disorders in older p. the expert consensus guideline series. pharmacotherapy of depressive disorders in older patients. Postgrad Med 2001;Spec No Pharmacotherapy:1–86.
45. Sajatovic M, Chen P. Geriatric bipolar disorder. Psychiatr Clin North Am 2011; 34(2):319–33, vii.
46. Young RC, Mulsant BH, Sajatovic M, et al. GERI-BD: A randomized double-blind controlled trial of lithium and divalproex in the treatment of mania in older patients with bipolar disorder. Am J Psychiatry 2017;174(11):1086–93.
47. Pollock BG, Mulsant BH, Rosen J, et al. Comparison of citalopram, perphenazine, and placebo for the acute treatment of psychosis and behavioral disturbances in hospitalized, demented patients. Am J Psychiatry 2002;159(3):460–5.
48. Pollock BG, Mulsant BH, Rosen J, et al. A double-blind comparison of citalopram and risperidone for the treatment of behavioral and psychotic symptoms associated with dementia. Am J Geriatr Psychiatry 2007;15(11):942–52.
49. Porsteinsson AP, Drye LT, Pollock BG, et al. Effect of citalopram on agitation in Alzheimer disease: the CitAD randomized clinical trial. JAMA 2014;311(7): 682–91.
50. Leonpacher AK, Peters ME, Drye LT, et al. Effects of Citalopram on Neuropsychiatric Symptoms in Alzheimer's Dementia: Evidence From the CitAD Study. Am J Psychiatry 2016;173(5):473–80.
51. Ehrhardt S, Porsteinsson AP, Munro CA, et al. Escitalopram for agitation in Alzheimer's disease (S-CitAD): Methods and design of an investigator-initiated, randomized, controlled, multicenter clinical trial. Alzheimers Dement 2019;15(11): 1427–36.
52. Schneider LS, Tariot PN, Dagerman KS, et al. Effectiveness of atypical antipsychotic drugs in patients with Alzheimer's disease. N Engl J Med 2006;355(15): 1525–38.
53. Sultzer DL, Davis SM, Tariot PN, et al. Clinical symptom responses to atypical antipsychotic medications in Alzheimer's disease: phase 1 outcomes from the CATIE-AD effectiveness trial. Am J Psychiatry 2008;165(7):844–54.
54. Yunusa I, Alsumali A, Garba AE, et al. Assessment of reported comparative effectiveness and safety of atypical antipsychotics in the treatment of behavioral and psychological symptoms of dementia: a network meta-analysis. JAMA Netw Open 2019;2(3):e190828.
55. Tariot PN, Cummings JL, Soto-Martin ME, et al. Trial of pimavanserin in dementia-related psychosis. N Engl J Med 2021;385(4):309–19.

56. PsychRights. FDA public health advisory deaths with antipsychotics in elderly patients with behavioral disturbance. 2022. Available at: http://psychrights.org/drugs/FDAantipsychotics4elderlywarning.htm. Accessed February 20, 2022.

57. Devanand DP, Crocco E, Forester BP, et al. Low dose lithium treatment of behavioral complications in alzheimer's disease: lit-ad randomized clinical trial. Am J Geriatr Psychiatry 2022;30(1):32–42.

58. Hu B, Ross L, Neuhaus J, et al. Off-label medication use in frontotemporal dementia. Am J Alzheimers Dis Other Demen 2010;25(2):128–33.

59. Riedl L, Mackenzie IR, Forstl H, et al. Frontotemporal lobar degeneration: current perspectives. Neuropsychiatr Dis Treat 2014;10:297–310.

60. Hall D, Finger EC. Psychotic symptoms in frontotemporal dementia. Curr Neurol Neurosci Rep 2015;15(7):46.

61. Thomsen TR, Panisset M, Suchowersky O, et al. Impact of standard of care for psychosis in Parkinson disease. J Neurol Neurosurg Psychiatry 2008;79(12):1413–5.

62. Chang A, Fox SH. Psychosis in Parkinson's Disease: Epidemiology, Pathophysiology, and Management. Drugs 2016;76(11):1093–118.

63. Friedman JH. Pharmacological interventions for psychosis in Parkinson's disease patients. Expert Opin Pharmacother 2018;19(5):499–505.

64. Voon V, Fox S, Butler TR, et al. Antidepressants and psychosis in Parkinson disease: a case series. Int J Geriatr Psychiatry 2007;22(6):601–4.

65. Watts KE, Storr NJ, Barr PG, et al. Systematic review of pharmacological interventions for people with Lewy body dementia. Aging Ment Health 2022;1–14.

66. McKeith I, Fairbairn A, Perry R, et al. Neuroleptic sensitivity in patients with senile dementia of Lewy body type. BMJ 1992;305(6855):673–8.

Substance Use Disorders in the Elderly

Rajesh R. Tampi, MD, MS, DFAPA, DFAAGP[a,b,*], Deena J. Tampi, MSN, MBA-HCA, RN, DFAAGP[c], Alisandrea Elson, MD[a]

KEYWORDS

- Substance use disorders • Elderly • Older adults • Alcohol • Tobacco • Cannabis
- Naltrexone

KEY POINTS

- Substance use disorders are not uncommon among the elderly.
- Substance use disorders are often underdiagnosed among the elderly.
- Substance use disorders result in worse outcomes among the elderly.
- The screening for substance use disorders among the elderly should occur during all routine medical appointments.
- The elderly with substance use disorders respond to treatment as well as younger adults with substance use disorders.

INTRODUCTION

The population of elderly (aged ≥65 years) in the United States is growing steadily. The number of older adults in the United States is expected to increase from 16.9% of the population in 2020 to 22% by 2050.[1] It is estimated that by 2034, there will be more elderly in the United States than children younger than 18 years (77 million vs 76.7 million).[2]

The *Diagnostic and Statistical Manual of Mental Disorders, Fifth Edition*, defines substance use disorder (SUD) as a problematic pattern of substance use that leads to clinically significant impairment or distress that is manifested by at least 2 of the following criteria occurring within a 12-month period.[3] These criteria include (1) the substance is taken in larger amounts or over a longer period than intended; (2) there is a persistent desire or unsuccessful efforts to cut down or control substance use; (3) a great deal of time is spent in activities to obtain substances, use them, or recover from their effects;

[a] Department of Psychiatry, Creighton University Education Building, 7710 Mercy Road, Suite 601, Omaha, NE 68124, USA; [b] Department of Psychiatry, Yale School of Medicine, 333 Cedar Street, New Haven, CT 06510, USA; [c] Behavioral Health Advisory Group, 259 Nassau Street, Suite2 #386, Princeton, NJ 08542, USA
* Corresponding author.
E-mail address: rajesh.tampi@gmail.com

Psychiatr Clin N Am 45 (2022) 707–716
https://doi.org/10.1016/j.psc.2022.07.005
0193-953X/22/© 2022 Elsevier Inc. All rights reserved.

(4) craving or a strong desire or urge to use a substance; (5) recurrent use of substance resulting in failure to fulfill major role obligations at work, school, or home; (6) continued use of the substance despite persistent or recurrent social or interpersonal problems caused or exacerbated by their effects; (7) important social, occupational, or recreational activities are given up or reduced because of substance use; (8) recurrent substance use in situations in which it is physically hazardous; (9) substance use is continued despite knowledge of having a persistent or recurrent physical or psychological problem that is likely to have been caused or exacerbated by drug use; (10) tolerance as defined by either a need for markedly increased amounts of the substance to achieve intoxication or desired effect or a markedly diminished effect with continued use of the same amount of the substance; and (11) withdrawal is manifested by either characteristic withdrawal symptoms or by the use of the substance (or a closely related substance) to relieve or avoid withdrawal symptoms.

In the United States the population of elderly with SUDs is increasing rapidly.[4] At present, there are about 5.7 million elderly individuals with SUDs in the United States[5]; this is a significant increase from 2006 when there were approximately 2.8 million elderly adults in the United States with SUDs. Health-related issues that are associated with aging and psychosocial stressors faced by these individuals can increase their exposure to psychoactive drugs, thus making the elderly an at-risk population for using these drugs.[6,7] Available evidence indicates that approximately 25% of the elderly have used a psychoactive drug that has a potential for misuse or abuse. The next section discusses specific substances of abuse among the elderly.

SUBSTANCES ABUSED BY THE ELDERLY

When compared with younger adults who tend to abuse marijuana, cocaine, and heroin, the elderly abuse alcohol, nicotine, and prescription medications.[6]

Alcohol

Alcohol is the substance that is most commonly used and misused by older adults.[8] Available evidence indicates that approximately 50% of individuals aged 65 years or older and about 25% individuals aged 85 years or older use alcohol.[9] Recent data indicate that 10.7% of elderly are engaged in past-month binge alcohol use, whereas 2.8% were engaged in past-month heavy alcohol use.[8] One national survey found that among the elderly, symptoms of alcohol abuse or dependence were noted among 6.7% of the individuals.[10] Another national survey found that among the elderly, 13% of men and 8% of women reported at-risk use of alcohol.[11] Binge drinking was reported among 14% of men and 3% of women in this group. The risk factors for binge drinking among these individuals were the concurrent use of tobacco and illicit drugs. In addition, individuals involved in binge drinking when compared with those individuals who did not use alcohol had higher incomes and were more often men. Furthermore, they had higher rates of being separated, divorced, or widowed. It was also noted in this study that African American women when compared with Caucasian women had a relatively high rate of binge drinking (10% vs 6%). Alcohol use disorder is also noted among 30% of the elderly who are admitted to medical units and in approximately 50% of the elderly admitted to psychiatric units.[9]

Tobacco

Past-year tobacco use is noted in 14.1% of elderly when compared with 30.2% of individuals aged 50 to 64 years.[12] Risk factors for cigarette use among older individuals include lower income levels, not being married, binge drinking, and the use of illicit and nonmedical drugs.

Marijuana, Cocaine, Stimulants, Hallucinogens, and Heroin

It is estimated that currently 5.1% of the elderly engage in past-year cannabis use.[8] Past-year cocaine use is seen in 0.04% of the elderly.[13] The past-year use rates of inhalants, hallucinogens, methamphetamine, and heroin is less than 0.2% among the elderly. Risk factors for marijuana use include male gender, being separated, being divorced or widowed, never being married, and a past-year history of major depressive disorder. Risk factors for cocaine use include male gender, being of Native American or of black decent, being unemployed, being separated, being divorced or widowed, having never-married status, and a past-year history of major depressive disorder.

Opioids

The past-year nonmedical use of prescription opioids (1.4%) among older individuals has been found to be more prevalent than nonmedical use of prescription sedatives (0.14%), tranquilizers (0.46%), and stimulants (0.16%).[14] Among older individuals, the past-year prevalence of prescription opioid use disorders is relatively low at 0.13%, but among nonmedical opioid users, the risk of prescription opioid dependence is fairly high at 7.6%.

Benzodiazepines

Approximately 15% of the elderly have used benzodiazepines in any given year.[15] Among the elderly, past-year benzodiazepine dependence is found in 3.3% of women and 0.8% of men living in the community.[16] Risk factors for benzodiazepine dependence in the elderly include female sex, having cognitive impairment, having panic disorder, having suicidal ideation, and feeling embarrassment in obtaining help for emotional problems.[17]

CHANGES IN SUBSTANCE USE PATTERNS AMONG THE ELDERLY

Available evidence indicates that the proportion of admissions due to alcohol use disorders as the primary substance of abuse has decreased from 84.7% to 75.9%, but the proportion of admissions due to opioids/heroin has increased from 6.6% to 10.5%.[18] During the same period, admissions due to cocaine use have doubled (2.1% to 4.4%) and admissions due to sedative use have tripled (0.5% to 1.3%).

Older adults often had no prior treatment episodes (36.9% vs 43.2%) and had used only one substance at admission (46% vs 77.1%) when compared with younger individuals.[19] In addition, a lower proportion of older individuals also reported using opioids/heroin (14.3% vs 21.1%) and cocaine/crack (5.4% vs 16.8%) when compared with younger individuals.

RISK FACTORS

The risk for SUDs is increased among the elderly who have prior history of substance use, among those individuals with comorbid psychiatric disorders and among those individuals with cognitive impairment.[14,20] Additional risk factors include being male, being Caucasian, having overall poor health status, having multiple comorbidities, having chronic pain, having disability or mobility issues, polypharmacy, unexpected retirement, bereavement, changes in living situation, and social isolation.[4] Being married, having no prior history of substance use, and having a religious affiliation are all considered to be mitigating factors for SUDs among the elderly.[13,14,21] SUDs are moderately to highly heritable, with heritability rates that range from 0.39 for hallucinogens to 0.72 for cocaine.[22]

CONSEQUENCES

Among older adults with SUD, worse medical outcomes and greater economic burden for care are noted.[6] In the elderly, the prolonged use of psychoactive substances can result in central nervous system adverse effects including drowsiness, confusion, impaired psychomotor activity, reduced reaction time, poor coordination, ataxia, falls, and amnesia, even at therapeutic doses.[23] Sustained use of these substances can result in physiologic dependence with withdrawal symptoms occurring if these substances are abruptly discontinued. In addition, the use of these substances can result in significant drug-drug interactions and adverse effects when they are used in conjunction with other prescribed medications or with over-the-counter drugs.[6]

Substance abuse in the elderly can result in multiple medical disorders, including cardiac, hepatic, and renal diseases, at rates higher than in younger patients.[24] Available evidence indicates that substance abuse in the elderly results in significant disability, morbidity, and mortality rates.[25]

Comorbid conditions are not uncommon in older adults with SUDs. One study found that approximately one-fifth of hospitalized older adults with psychiatric disorders had a comorbid substance abuse disorder.[26] Another study evaluating older adults who were receiving outpatient care found that most of these individuals (>90%) had comorbid SUDs.[27] One study found that men with a history of heavy drinking for 5 years or more at some time in their lives have a greater than 5-fold risk of suffering from a psychiatric disorder.[28] Older adults with SUDs have higher rates of depression and suicides than age-matched controls.[29,30]

The overall cost of SUDs in the United States is estimated to be greater than US $100 billion per year.[23] Available data indicate that the economic costs associated with SUDs in late life is high due to greater morbidity and potentially more serious health problems in this age group. Also, these individuals have longer inpatient hospital lengths of stay and need more outpatient visits to manage their symptoms when compared with age-matched controls.[31,32]

ASSESSMENT

Available evidence indicates that among the elderly, SUDs are often underdiagnosed.[23] Denial of the condition, stigma and/or shame of using addictive substances, reluctance to seek professional help, the lack of financial resources and/or social supports, along with insufficient knowledge of SUDs among older individuals are often cited as barriers to appropriate identification and treatment of these disorders. Often, inaccurate diagnosis of SUDs among the elderly occurs due to the ageist attitudes toward psychiatric disorders among these individuals, the presence of comorbid disorders, and the limited time that health care providers spend with the older individuals.

Among the elderly, the signs and symptoms of SUDs may be difficult to recognize because the standard diagnostic criteria used to identify SUDs among the adult population have not been validated among the older individuals.[4,7,33] These criteria often underestimate the prevalence of SUDs among the elderly.[7,33] Body changes due to the aging process alters the body's ability to develop tolerance to drugs.[34] Older adults may demonstrate greater substance-related problems, even though their patterns of use have remained stable. Also, age-related physiologic changes can enhance the effects of tolerance and withdrawal, leading to protracted symptoms.[7]

It may also be difficult for the elderly to recall the details of their substance use due to cognitive decline.[7] Because there are often age-appropriate changes in social roles among the elderly, the negative effect of SUDs on their social life may be less prominent among these individuals.[7] Also, the detection of impairments in social roles due to SUDs may be difficult because many older individuals may be less active in their social life.[34] The presence of comorbid illnesses and changes in the body due to the aging process may provide confounders to or may mask signs and symptoms of SUDs, including memory difficulties or falls.[24]

The Treatment Improvement Protocol (TIP) consensus panel recommends that health care providers screen for alcohol, tobacco, prescription drug, and illicit drug use in all older clients at least annually.[35] It would be prudent for these screenings to be conducted by primary care providers because the elderly are more commonly evaluated by their primary care providers for medical issues, rather than mental health providers or other specialists.[36] Evidence indicates that the identification and treatment of SUDs in the elderly has improved due to the presence of community-based programs for screening and brief interventions for these disorders.[37]

The identification of SUDs in the elderly can be improved by the use of validated screening tools.[24] It is recommended that screening for SUDs among the elderly should be conducted regularly, especially before starting new medications and/or when potential substance-related problems have arisen, including injuries or accidents.[35] The screening instruments could be administered as part of an interview or as a part of other health screenings. Screening tools that can be used among the elderly with SUDs include (1) alcohol: Alcohol Use Disorders Identification Test (AUDIT), Alcohol Use Disorders Identification Test-C (AUDIT-C), Short Michigan Alcoholism Screening Test-Geriatric Version (SMAST-G), and the Senior Alcohol Misuse Indicator (SAMI); (2) cannabis: Cannabis Use Disorder Identification Test-Revised (CUDIT-R); and (3) multiple substances: Alcohol, Smoking, and Substance Involvement Screening Test (ASSIST), Brief Addiction Monitor, CAGE Adapted to Include Drugs (CAGE-AID), and the National Institute on Drug Abuse (NIDA) Quick Screen V1.0. In primary care settings, computerized screening tools such as the Drug and Alcohol Problem Assessment for Primary Care (DAPA-PC) has been useful in identifying and managing SUDs among the elderly.[36,38] **Fig. 1** describes the assessment of the elderly with SUDs.[39]

TREATMENTS

Available evidence indicates that elderly with SUDs respond to treatment as well as younger individuals with SUDs.[40,41] Treatment response seems to be better among older women and with longer duration of treatment.[42] It has also been noted that

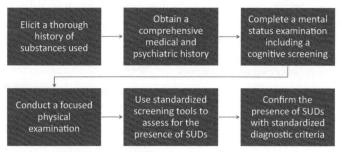

Fig. 1. Assessment of elderly with SUDs.[39]

specialized treatment programs for older adults with SUDs have shown greater benefits because many of these individuals have comorbidities and age-related health care changes when compared with younger individuals.[6,43] Inpatient level of care where there is closer monitoring of health care needs, including drug interactions and side effects of treatments, may often be more appropriate for the elderly with SUDs.[6,43]

The TIPS consensus panel recommends that all treatments for SUDs among the elderly should be provided using age-sensitive practices.[35] These include treatment modalities that should be supportive, nonconfrontational, flexible, and sensitive to gender and cultural differences.[7] Brief intervention strategies and motivational counseling should be considered as initial steps in the treatment of SUDs in the elderly.[23] Specialized treatment programs should be reserved for individuals who fail less intensive treatments. Treatment strategies that are more successful among the elderly often address age-specific medical, psychological, and social issues.[7]

Cognitive behavioral approaches, individual counseling, group-based treatments, marital and family involvement/family therapy, medical/psychiatric treatments, case management, community-linked services, and outreach programs are recommended treatments for older individuals with SUD.[23] Better outcomes are also noted when there is provision of age-specific treatments, the use of age-appropriate pace and content, and the use of supportive and nonconfrontational approaches that build self-esteem.[7,23] In addition, benefits are also noted when there is development of skills that improve social supports. Older adults also find benefit with the use of counselors who are specialized in working with this age group.

Screening, Brief Intervention, and Referral to Treatment (SBIRT) is an evidence-based approach to managing individuals who exhibit at-risk drug use, misuse of prescription medications, or use illicit substances.[35] SBIRT has also been found to be beneficial among older adults, and it can be applied to nonmedical services that serve this age group.[44] **Fig. 2** describes the pathway for the treatment of elderly individuals with SUDs.[35]

Owing to physiologic changes associated with aging, withdrawal symptoms from alcohol and other substances of abuse may often be more intense and prolonged among the elderly.[6,43] Older individuals who are acutely intoxicated and those individuals who are in acute withdrawal should have medical stabilization and supervised medical withdrawal substances. Acute inpatient treatment may also be required for older individuals who are frail, use multiple substances, have used high doses of alcohol or drugs, and have active suicidal ideation/plan.

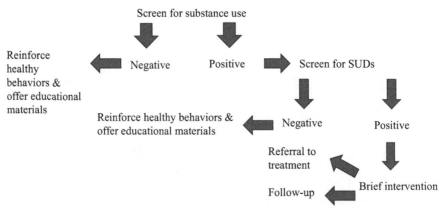

Fig. 2. Treatment of SUDs in the elderly.[35]

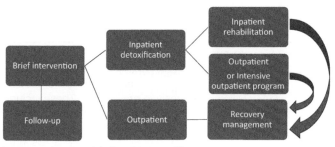

Fig. 3. Levels of care for the elderly with SUDs.[35]

In the United States, the Food and Drug Administration has approved acamprosate, disulfiram, and naltrexone for the treatment of alcohol use disorder and buprenorphine for the treatment of opioid use disorder among adults; however, the data on the use of these medications from controlled trials for the treatment of SUDs among older adults are limited.[45] A review of the literature indicates that there are only 2 randomized controlled trials that evaluated the use of pharmacologic agents for SUDs among the older individuals (≥50 years). In 1 trial, naltrexone was compared with placebo for the treatment of alcohol use disorder among individuals aged 50 to 70 years. In the second trial, naltrexone or placebo was used as adjunct with sertraline for the treatment of alcohol use disorder among individuals aged 55 years or older. In both trials, the use of naltrexone reduced the rates of relapse among the older individuals with alcohol use disorder. The search did not identify any controlled trials of buprenorphine, acamprosate, or disulfiram among the elderly with SUDs.

Once the elderly individual has completed treatment of SUDs, they should be provided with recovery management.[35] Recovery management describes the organizing philosophy for the treatment of SUDs and recovery support services that assist the individual and their family members achieve and maintain sustained recovery. The individuals who are most likely to benefit from recovery management include those elderly with co-occurring medical conditions or mental disorders, those who are socially isolated, and those individuals who have limited support from family and friends. Interventions that have shown to benefit in recovery management among the elderly include home visits, telephone counseling, recovery checkups, linkages to community resources including recovery support groups, and using case management services. **Fig. 3** describes the levels of care for elderly with SUDs.[35]

SUMMARY

SUDs are not uncommon among the elderly. These disorders are often missed among the elderly for multiple reasons. One reason is that the standardized diagnostic criteria are less sensitive in identifying SUDs among the elderly when compared with younger individuals. The routine screening for SUDs among older adults, along with the use of validated screening tools will improve the identification of these disorders among older adults. The treatment of SUDs among the elderly indicates that specialized programs that are sensitive to the needs of the older individuals have more success than general SUD programs. Many older individuals with SUDs do not need referrals to specialized treatment programs. Using evidence-based models like SBIRT will assist with identifying and referring only those older individuals who need specialized care to these more intensive programs. Although the data for the pharmacologic treatment of SUDs from controlled trials are limited, available data indicate that older adults with SUDs respond well to treatments.

CLINICS CARE POINTS

- The population of elderly with SUDs in the United States is growing.
- SUDs among the elderly are often underdiagnosed.
- SUDs among the elderly are associated with poor outcomes.
- Currently available diagnostic criteria are less sensitive in identifying SUDs among the elderly.
- The use of routine screening with validated screening tools may improve diagnosis of SUDs among the elderly.
- Data on the pharmacologic treatment of SUDs among the elderly from controlled studies is limited.
- Elderly with SUDs respond well to treatments that are specifically designed for this age group.

DISCLOSURE

The authors have no relevant affiliations or financial involvement with any organization or entity with a financial interest in or financial conflict with the subject matter or materials discussed in the article, including employment, consultancies, honoraria, stock ownership or options, expert testimony, grants or patents received or pending, or royalties. No writing assistance was used in the production of this article.

REFERENCES

1. Share of old age population (65 years and older) in the total U.S. population from 1950 to 2050. Available at: https://www.statista.com/statistics/457822/share-of-old-age-population-in-the-total-us-population/. Accessed January 23, 2022.
2. The U.S. Joins Other Countries With Large Aging Populations. Available at: https://www.census.gov/library/stories/2018/03/graying-america.html. Accessed January 23, 2022.
3. Diagnostic and Statistical Manual of Mental Disorders. Substance-Related and Addictive Disorders. Available at: https://doi.org/10.1176/appi.books.9780890425596.dsm16. Accessed February 12, 2022.
4. Kuerbis A, Sacco P, Blazer DG, et al. Substance abuse among older adults. Clin Geriatr Med 2014;30(3):629-654.
5. Yarnell S, Li L, MacGrory B, et al. Substance Use Disorders in Later Life: A Review and Synthesis of the Literature of an Emerging Public Health Concern. Am J Geriatr Psychiatry 2020;28(2):226-36.
6. Simoni-Wastila L, Yang HK. Psychoactive drug abuse in older adults. Am J Geriatr Pharmacother 2006;4(4):380-94.
7. Wu LT, Blazer DG. Illicit and nonmedical drug use among older adults: a review. J Aging Health 2011;23(3):481-504.
8. Center for Behavioral Health Statistics and Quality. Results from the 2019 national survey on drug use and health: detailed tables. Rockville, MD: Substance Abuse and Mental Health Services Administration; 2020. Available at: https://www.samhsa.gov/data/. Accessed February 3, 2022.
9. Caputo F, Vignoli T, Leggio L, et al. Alcohol use disorders in the elderly: A brief overview from epidemiology to treatment options. Exp Gerontol 2012;47(6):411-6.

10. Blazer DG, Wu LT. The epidemiology of alcohol use disorders and subthreshold dependence in a middle-aged and elderly community sample. Am J Geriatr Psychiatry 2011;19(8):685–94.

11. Blazer DG, Wu LT. The epidemiology of at-risk and binge drinking among middle-aged and elderly community adults: National Survey on Drug Use and Health. Am J Psychiatry 2009;166(10):1162–9.

12. Blazer DG, Wu LT. Patterns of tobacco use and tobacco-related psychiatric morbidity and substance use among middle-aged and older adults in the United States. Aging Ment Health 2012;16(3):296–304.

13. Blazer DG, Wu LT. The epidemiology of substance use and disorders among middle aged and elderly community adults: national survey on drug use and health. Am J Geriatr Psychiatry 2009;17(3):237–45.

14. Blazer DG, Wu LT. Nonprescription use of pain relievers by middle-aged and elderly community-living adults: National Survey on Drug Use and Health. J Am Geriatr Soc 2009;57(7):1252–7.

15. Llorente MD, David D, Golden AG, et al. Defining patterns of benzodiazepine use in older adults. J Geriatr Psychiatry Neurol 2000;13(3):150–60.

16. Préville M, Boyer R, Grenier S, et al. The epidemiology of psychiatric disorders in Quebec's older adult population. Can J Psychiatry 2008;53(12):822–32.

17. Voyer P, Préville M, Roussel ME, et al. Factors associated with benzodiazepine dependence among community-dwelling seniors. J Community Health Nurs 2009;26(3):101–13.

18. Substance Abuse and Mental Health Services Administration. The DASIS Report: Adults Aged 65 or Older in Substance Abuse Treatment: 2005. Rockville, MD: Substance Abuse and Mental Health Services Administration (SAMHSA); 2007.

19. Arndt S, Gunter TD, Acion L. Older admissions to substance abuse treatment in 2001. Am J Geriatr Psychiatry 2005;13(5):385–92.

20. Voyer P, Préville M, Cohen D, et al. The prevalence of benzodiazepine dependence among community-dwelling older adult users in Quebec according to typical and atypical criteria. Can J Aging 2010;29(2):205–13.

21. Han B, Gfroerer JC, Colliver JD. An examination of trends in illicit drug use among adults aged 50 to 59 in the United States. Rockville, MD: Office of Applied Studies; 2009.

22. Bevilacqua L, Goldman D. Genes and addictions. Clin Pharmacol Ther 2009; 85(4):359–61.

23. Cook P, Davis C, Howard DL, et al. Substance Abuse among Older Adults. Treatment Improvement Protocol (TIP) Series 26. Published online 1998.

24. Dowling GJ, Weiss SRB, Condon TP. Drugs of abuse and the gaining brain. Neuropsychopharmacology 2008;33:209–18.

25. Reid MC, Anderson PA. Geriatric substance use disorders. Med Clin North Am 1997;81(4):999–1016.

26. Whitcup SM, Miller F. Unrecognized drug dependence in psychiatrically hospitalized elderly patients. J Am Geriatr Soc 1987;35(4):297–301.

27. Holroyd S, Duryee JJ. Substance use disorders in a geriatric psychiatry outpatient clinic: prevalence and epidemiologic characteristics. J Nerv Ment Dis 1997;185(10):627–32.

28. Saunders PA, Copeland JR, Dewey ME, et al. Heavy drinking as a risk factor for depression and dementia in elderly men. Findings from the Liverpool longitudinal community study. Br J Psychiatry 1991;159:213–6.

29. Blow FC, Brockmann LM, Barry KL. Role of alcohol in late-life suicide. Alcohol Clin Exp Res 2004;28(5 Suppl):48S–56S.

30. Blow FC, Serras AM, Barry KL. Late-life depression and alcoholism. Curr Psychiatry Rep 2007;9(1):14–9.
31. Prigerson HG, Desai RA, Rosenheck RA. Older adult patients with both psychiatric and substance abuse disorders: prevalence and health service use. Psychiatr Q 2001;72(1):1–18.
32. Brennan PL, Nichols KA, Moos RH. Long-term use of VA mental health services by older patients with substance use disorders. Psychiatr Serv 2002;53(7): 836–41.
33. Patterson TL, Jeste DV. The potential impact of the baby-boom generation on substance abuse among elderly persons. Psychiatr Serv 1999;50(9):1184–8.
34. Fingerhood M. Substance abuse in older people. J Am Geriatr Soc 2000;48(8): 985–95.
35. Treating Substance Use Disorder in Older Adults: UPDATED 2020. Substance Abuse and Mental Health Services Administration (US); 2020. Available at: http://www.ncbi.nlm.nih.gov/books/NBK571029/. Accessed February 12, 2022.
36. Nemes S, Rao PA, Zeiler C, et al. Computerized screening of substance abuse problems in a primary care setting: older vs. younger adults. Am J Drug Alcohol Abuse 2004;30(3):627–42.
37. Schonfeld L, King-Kallimanis BL, Duchene DM, et al. Screening and brief intervention for substance misuse among older adults: the Florida BRITE project. Am J Public Health 2010;100(1):108–14.
38. Holtz K, Landis R, Nemes S, et al. Development of a computerized screening system to identify substance abuse in primary care. J Healthc Qual 2001;23(3): 34–7, 45.
39. Introduction to the Canadian Coalition for Seniors' Mental Health (CCSMH) Guidelines on Substance Use Disorders Among Older Adults. Available at: https://ccsmh.ca/wp-content/uploads/2019/12/Canadian_Guidelines_Introduction_Doc_ENG.pdf. Accessed February 12, 2022.
40. Blow FC, Walton MA, Chermack ST, et al. Older adult treatment outcome following elder-specific inpatient alcoholism treatment. J Subst Abuse Treat 2000;19(1): 67–75.
41. Satre DD, Mertens JR, Areán PA, et al. Five-year alcohol and drug treatment outcomes of older adults versus middle-aged and younger adults in a managed care program. Addiction 2004;99(10):1286–97.
42. Satre DD, Blow FC, Chi FW, et al. Gender differences in seven-year alcohol and drug treatment outcomes among older adults. Am J Addict 2007;16(3):216–21.
43. Menninger JA. Assessment and treatment of alcoholism and substance-related disorders in the elderly. Bull Menninger Clin 2002;66(2):166–83.
44. Schonfeld L, Hazlett RW, Hedgecock DK, et al. Gum AM. Screening, Brief Intervention, and Referral to Treatment for Older Adults With Substance Misuse. Am J Public Health 2015;105(1):205–11.
45. Tampi RR, Chhatlani A, Ahmad H, et al. Substance use disorders among older adults: A review of randomized controlled pharmacotherapy trials. World J Psychiatry 2019;9(5):78–82.

Insomnia and Other Sleep Disorders in Older Adults

Zachary L. Cohen, MD[a],*, Paul M. Eigenberger, MD[b],
Katherine M. Sharkey, MD, PhD[c,d], Michelle L. Conroy, MD[b,e],
Kirsten M. Wilkins, MD[b,e]

KEYWORDS

- Geriatric psychiatry • Geriatrics • Insomnia • Sleep disorders
- Age-related changes in sleep • Treatment of insomnia • CBT-I

KEY POINTS

- Sleep disturbances are associated with many poor health outcomes in older adults, including increased risk for falls, cognitive decline, and all-cause mortality.
- Insomnia is often related to underlying medical, psychiatric, or environmental factors. A thorough medical and psychiatric history and an understanding of sleep environment and psychosocial stressors are essential when evaluating sleep disturbances.
- Many medications can cause or contribute to insomnia and other sleep disorders. It is critical to review patients' medication lists and if feasible, discontinue or reduce the dosages of agents that may be contributing to sleep disturbances.
- Cognitive behavioral therapy for insomnia is the first-line treatment for adults with chronic insomnia and is available in many different modalities.
- Benzodiazepines, "Z-drugs," and significantly anticholinergic medications such as diphenhydramine should be avoided in older adults. Providers should carefully weigh the potential adverse events and side effects of agents that do have evidence for effective use in older adults.

Abbreviations	
CBT-I	Cognitive Behavioral Therapy for Insomnia

[a] Department of Psychiatry, University of North Carolina at Chapel Hill, 101 Manning Drive, Campus Box #7160, Chapel Hill, NC, 27599, USA; [b] Yale University School of Medicine, 300 George Street, Suite #901, New Haven, CT, 06511, USA; [c] Department of Medicine, The Warren Alpert Medical School of Brown University, 233 Richmond Street, Suite 242, Providence, RI 02903, USA; [d] Department of Psychiatry and Human Behavior, The Warren Alpert Medical School of Brown University, 233 Richmond Street, Suite 242, Providence, RI 02903, USA; [e] VA Connecticut Healthcare System, West Haven, CT, USA
* Corresponding author.
E-mail address: zachary_cohen@med.unc.edu

Psychiatr Clin N Am 45 (2022) 717–734
https://doi.org/10.1016/j.psc.2022.07.002
0193-953X/22/© 2022 Elsevier Inc. All rights reserved.
psych.theclinics.com

INTRODUCTION

Approximately half of older adults (typically defined as age 65 years and older) report sleep disturbances.[1,2] Several common sleep disorders are more prevalent in older adults than in younger individuals. This increased prevalence is associated with various correlates of aging, including sleep architecture changes, medical, psychiatric and neurocognitive diseases, untreated or undertreated pain, medication side effects, and stressors such as social isolation, racial discrimination, bereavement, and caregiving responsibilities.[3–6]

Sleep disturbances are associated with poor health outcomes in older adults, including increased fall risk, higher rates of depression, poorer control of chronic medical conditions, greater morbidity from acute medical illness, increased risk for cognitive decline, and increased all-cause mortality, even after controlling for factors such as medication use, age, mobility, and baseline health status.[3,7–12] In other words, sleep disturbances may not only be symptoms of medical, psychiatric, and neurocognitive disorders but may also be risk factors for developing or worsening these conditions.[3,13]

With the worldwide population of people aged 65 or older projected to more than double from 727 million in 2020 to over 1.5 billion in 2050, sleep symptoms will be encountered by many providers with increasing frequency.[14] It is vital for those who care for older adults to understand age-related sleep changes and have a framework for prevention, diagnosis, and treatment of insomnia and other disorders that impact this population so significantly.

Although insomnia is the primary focus of this article, the authors also review other sleep disorders that are more prevalent in older age, some of which are associated with cognitive impairment and/or neurodegenerative disorders. These include advanced sleep–wake phase disorder (ASWPD), rapid eye movement (REM) sleep behavior disorder (RBD), obstructive sleep apnea (OSA), restless leg syndrome (RLS), and periodic limb movement disorder (PLMD).[15–18]

AGE-RELATED CHANGES IN SLEEP AND CIRCADIAN RHYTHMS

Developmental changes in sleep occur throughout the lifespan, and older adults experience normal, age-related changes in sleep and circadian rhythms.[19] Sleep architecture refers to the classification of sleep into different stages, as measured by brain wave patterns, eye movements, and muscle tone.[20] Sleep consists of three non-REM stages known as N1, N2, and N3 and REM sleep.[20,21] Compared with younger persons, older adults spend more time in N1 and N2, the "shallow" stages of sleep in which awakenings can occur more readily, and less time in stage N3 (deep, slow-wave sleep) and REM sleep[22–24] (**Box 1**).

The National Sleep Foundation recommends 7 to 8 hours of sleep for older adults, similar to the 7 to 9 hours recommended for those under age 65 years.[25] Evidence suggests that older adults who sleep between 6 and 9 hours have improved mental and physical health, cognition, and quality of life compared with those with shorter or longer durations.[4]

Sleep efficiency (SE)—defined as the percentage of time in bed spent sleeping compared with the total time spent in bed—continues to decrease after age 60.[19] This is particularly relevant to insomnia, as decreased SE essentially represents increased time spent in bed trying to fall and stay asleep. Improvement in SE is a key measure in evaluating the efficacy of insomnia treatment, and SE is used to implement sleep restriction therapy (SRT), a major component of cognitive behavioral

---

Box 1
Age-related changes in sleep and circadian rhythms

- Increased N1 sleep
- Increased N2 sleep
- Decreased N3 sleep
- Decreased REM sleep
- Earlier typical bedtimes
- Earlier circadian preference (greater "morningness")
- Shorter nighttime sleep duration
- Greater sleep fragmentation
- Increased time awake after sleep onset
- More frequent napping
- Decreased sleep efficiency

---

therapy for insomnia (CBT-I). Reduced SE has been associated with increased risk for falls, frailty, and death.[8,26,27]

The sleep–wake cycle changes with age. Circadian rhythms, intrinsic 24-hour cycles that govern the sleep–wake cycle and other physiologic processes, become less effective at responding to external cues or "zeitgebers" ("time givers" in German) that signal when one should sleep or wake, and thus the sleep–wake cycle becomes less consistent.[7] Many older adults have less exposure to these cues. For example, older adults, especially those who have Alzheimer's disease and/or live in institutional settings, have substantially less exposure to bright light, the strongest entrainer of circadian rhythms.[28] Further, dim light melatonin onset, the time at which the pineal gland releases endogenous melatonin in response to dim light, typically 2 to 3 hours before one's habitual bedtime, commonly occurs earlier in the day in healthy older adults. This can be accompanied by a "phase advanced" sleep–wake cycle, that is, the individual falls asleep earlier and wakes up earlier than is typical.[7,29–31] Older adults may also struggle to stay awake during the day and engage in more frequent napping, which can alter circadian rhythms.[13,32]

There are also sleep parameters that do not change significantly in older age. Total daily sleep duration decreases by about 10 minutes per every decade of life, but it does not decrease significantly past age 60. Sleep-onset latency, the amount of time it takes to transition from wakefulness to sleep, increases but only by approximately 10 minutes in total between the ages of 20 and 80, an effect that levels off by age 60.[19] Healthy older adults often have more frequent awakenings but they fall back asleep in a similar amount of time as their younger counterparts.[33]

INSOMNIA DISORDER

Insomnia is the most prevalent sleep disorder, and symptom burden increases with age, particularly for women.[15,34] Although insomnia can manifest as a primary disorder, it is frequently comorbid and multifactorial in origin (**Box 2**).[35] "Comorbid insomnia" refers to insomnia that is directly related to an underlying medical, psychiatric, or environmental cause.[36] A thorough medical and psychiatric history and an understanding of sleep environment and psychosocial stressors are essential when evaluating sleep disturbances **Box 2**.

> **Box 2**
> **The Diagnostic and Statistical Manual of Mental Disorders, Fifth Edition (DSM-5) criteria for insomnia disorder[15]**
>
> - Dissatisfaction with sleep quantity or quality, associated with one or more of the following:
>   - Difficulty initiating sleep
>   - Difficulty maintaining sleep—characterized by frequent awakenings or problems returning to sleep after awakenings
>   - Early morning awakening with inability to return to sleep
> - Clinically significant distress or functional impairment
> - Occurs at least three nights per week and be present for at least 3 months, despite adequate opportunity for sleep
> - Cannot be attributable to the physiologic effects of a substance nor be explained predominantly by a coexisting psychiatric or medical illness.

MEDICAL, PSYCHIATRIC, AND ENVIRONMENTAL FACTORS IMPACTING INSOMNIA AND OTHER SLEEP DISTURBANCES
Medical Comorbidities

The more comorbidities an older adult has, the more likely he or she is to report a sleep complaint.[37] Common medical conditions strongly associated with insomnia and reduced sleep quality include heart disease, cancer, hypertension, neurodegenerative disorders, respiratory disease (including OSA), urinary issues, diabetes, chronic pain, and gastrointestinal disorders.[38–40] When evaluating a sleep concern, clinicians should screen for shortness of breath, somatic pain, nocturia, gastrointestinal symptoms, and limitations in mobility, all of which may compromise sleep and should be addressed.[41]

The Effects of Medications on Sleep

Almost 40% of older adults take five or more prescription medications.[42] Many medications can cause, or contribute to, insomnia and other sleep disturbances, including RLS and RBD. **Table 1** shows an abbreviated list of common medications that may disturb sleep. The effects of withdrawal from medications may also interfere with sleep.

Medications with anticholinergic or antihistaminic properties, anticonvulsants, antispasmodics, benzodiazepines, and opiates can all cause daytime somnolence that can interfere with the sleep–wake cycle. Benzodiazepines and opiates can also worsen OSA, cause cognitive impairment, and increase fall risk.[43] These medications should be avoided in older adults whenever possible.

Providers should discontinue unnecessary medications and consider reducing the dosage of agents that may be contributing to sleep disturbance but are medically necessary. It is also important to avoid a prescribing cascade wherein medications such as hypnotics or stimulants are used to treat sleep-related side effects of other medications.[43] Reviewing the timing of medication administration is prudent; stimulating medications and diuretics should be taken as far from bedtime as possible, and sedating medications should be taken closer to bedtime.[28]

Psychiatric Conditions

Anxiety and depression are the most common psychiatric conditions in which older adults report difficulties with sleep onset or maintenance.[47] The association between insomnia and mood disorders is bidirectional; sleep disturbances can be both risk factors and consequences of anxiety and mood disorders. If left untreated, insomnia may

Table 1
Adverse sleep effects of medications commonly prescribed to older adults[4,28,43–46]

Medications	Effect(s) on Sleep	Possible Mechanism(s)
Beta-adrenergic blockers	Somnolence or insomnia	Vasodilatation through alpha-1 blockade (sedation); high beta-2 and 5-hydroxytryptamine receptor occupancy (insomnia); inhibition of melatonin production (insomnia)
Angiotensin-converting enzyme inhibitors	Insomnia	Cough
Angiotensin II receptor blockers	Insomnia	Unknown
Dopamine agonists	Somnolence (low doses) or insomnia (higher doses)	Dopamine agonism
Dopamine antagonists	RLS	
Antihistamines	RLS	
Melatonin	RLS	
Levothyroxine	Insomnia	Effects on hypothalamic-pituitary-adrenal axis; increasing histamine in hypothalamus and cerebral cortex
Loop diuretics	Insomnia	Nocturia
SSRIs/SNRIs	Daytime sedation, insomnia RLS RBD	Inhibition of serotonin and norepinephrine reuptake
Tricyclic antidepressants	RBD	
Mirtazapine	RBD Nightmares	
Psychostimulants (eg, methylphenidate)	Insomnia RLS	Sympathomimetic effects
Pseudoephedrine, ephedrine	Insomnia RLS	Sympathomimetic effects
Beta-agonists (inhaled and oral)	Insomnia	Sympathomimetic effects
Corticosteroids	Insomnia	Effects on hypothalamic-pituitary-adrenal axis; effects on cytokines

Abbreviations: RBD, rapid eye movement sleep behavior disorder; RLS, restless leg syndrome; SNRIs, serotonin and norepinephrine reuptake inhibitors; SSRIs, selective serotonin reuptake inhibitors.

also diminish treatment response to psychiatric illness and is associated with longer time to recovery, higher likelihood of relapse, higher health care utilization, and more frequent suicidal ideation.[48–50]

Other comorbid psychiatric conditions, notably bipolar affective disorder and post-traumatic stress disorder, are also strongly associated with sleep disturbances.[51,52]

Sleep Environment

Environmental factors such as noise, light, temperature, bedroom environment, disruptive medical care, social interaction, and sleep–wake patterns can all contribute to sleep disturbance.[43] The use of light-emitting devices such as smart phones, tablets, and e-readers before bed has been shown to alter circadian rhythms, which may potentiate poor sleep.[53]

Bereavement

The loss of a loved one is a common occurrence in older patients, and there is a strong relationship between bereavement and decreased sleep quality, especially with "complicated grief" or the DSM-5's persistent complex bereavement disorder, which is characterized by at least 12 months of clinically significant distress or functional impairment that is outside of sociocultural norms, in response to the death of a loved one. Grief therapy has been shown to partially improve sleep symptoms in bereavement.[54]

EVALUATION AND DIAGNOSIS
Taking a Sleep History

The evaluation of the older patient with sleep difficulties begins with gathering a thorough sleep, psychiatric, and medical history and should incorporate collateral information from a bed partner or caretaker if possible. A sleep history should identify chief sleep complaints, which commonly include one or more of the following: inability to fall asleep, inability to stay asleep, waking too early, poor sleep quality, too little sleep, work or lifestyle interfering with sleep, or inability to sleep without medications. The daytime consequences should be elicited.[55] Sleep-onset latency or time awake after sleep onset greater than 30 minutes is considered clinically significant in adults, although quantification is not necessary for diagnosis.[56]

An assessment of current sleep behaviors is the next task of a sleep history. This can be done retrospectively during a clinical interview, or prospectively with the use of a sleep diary, such as the Consensus Sleep Diary.[57] Pertinent data include bedtime, time the individual actively tries to fall asleep, sleep latency, wake time, time the individual gets out of bed to start the day, timing and number of nighttime awakenings, daytime naps, differences in weekday/weekend behavior, an inventory of prescription and over-the-counter (OTC) medications and their effectiveness, substance use (including alcohol, caffeine, nicotine, and other substances), presleep activities (e.g., use of electronics, exercise, food and liquid intake), perceived cause of insomnia (e.g., stress, nocturia, environmental factors), coping response to poor sleep, and factors that improve or worsen sleep.[55]

Drawing on collateral from a bed partner and/or caretaker, clinicians should assess for symptoms such as abnormal breathing and nocturnal movements that could be indicative of OSA, RLS, PLMD, or RBD.

Diagnosis

Many sleep disorders can be diagnosed clinically using DSM-5 criteria alone. However, several screening tools are practical supplements for assessment of sleep disturbances and can also be used to monitor treatment response. The Insomnia Severity Index consists of seven items that assess symptoms over the prior 2 weeks.[58] The Pittsburgh Sleep Quality Index measures seven domains of sleep over the prior month, yielding a global sleep quality score.[59] Either can typically be administered in 10 minutes or less. Another important and simple screening tool is the STOP-Bang questionnaire, which is used to stratify risk for OSA. It consists of eight yes/no items regarding clinical features of sleep apnea.[60]

In-laboratory polysomnography (PSG) or home sleep testing is not necessary to diagnosis insomnia but may be indicated when there is suspicion for another primary sleep disorder that may better explain the symptoms or a comorbid sleep disorder, such as OSA. PSG may also be indicated to assess for RBD or PMLD or when insomnia is refractory to treatment.[55]

TREATMENT OF INSOMNIA
Non-Pharmacological Interventions

Given the increased potential for adverse medication side effects in older adults, non-pharmacological interventions for insomnia are first line.[61] Behavioral approaches target thoughts, feelings, and behaviors that cause, perpetuate, and exacerbate poor sleep. They include sleep hygiene education (SHE), SRT, stimulus control therapy (SCT), relaxation techniques (RT), cognitive therapy (CT), and CBT-I. All have demonstrated sustained efficacy for older adults, including those with medical and psychiatric comorbidities.[62–64] Multimodal CBT-I combines several of these approaches. Mindfulness training is emerging as another evidence-based option for treating insomnia in older adults.[65]

Sleep Hygiene Education

Sleep hygiene education is the mostly widely disseminated behavioral treatment strategy, given its low resource intensity (**Box 3**). The drawback of SHE is that it is generally not efficacious as a stand-alone treatment of chronic insomnia and may delay the use of more effective treatment **Box 3**.[66]

Multimodal Cognitive Behavioral Therapy for Insomnia

The American College of Physicians endorses CBT-I as the first-line treatment for adults with chronic insomnia.[68] It has also been found to reduce concurrent depression and suicidality.[69] CBT-I consists of 6 to 10 sessions and includes components of SRT and SCT; it may also encompass SH, CT, and RT.

Box 3
Sleep hygiene recommendations[67]

- Avoid caffeine past noon
- Avoid naps past noon
- Avoid exercise within 2 hours of bedtime
- Avoid tobacco or nicotine products, especially within 2 hours of bedtime
- Avoid alcohol use, especially within 2 hours of bedtime
- Avoid heavy meals within 2 hours of bedtime
- Do not take over-the-counter sleep medications or supplements unless directed by a health care provider
- Go to sleep and wake up at the same time every day
- Maximize comfort of sleeping environment by controlling temperature and noise
- Avoid spending more than 20 minutes awake in bed; engage in an activity that does not involve a light-emitting device until sleepy, and then go back to bed

One barrier to CBT-I is a scarcity of trained clinicians to deliver individual treatment, which has resulted in the development of alternate delivery models such as group therapy, abridged protocols, and telephone, video, and application-based therapies. In older adults, the choice of CBT-I modality should weigh technology literacy, Internet access, and vision and hearing impairment, any of which could limit implementation.[66] However, a 2018 randomized placebo-controlled trial of Internet-based CBT found decreased rates of attrition with each decade above the study's average age of about 44 year old, diminishing the frequent assumption that older age limits one's ability to use digital CBT-I modalities.[70]

PHARMACOLOGIC TREATMENT OF INSOMNIA
General Principles

If non-pharmacological interventions for insomnia are not sufficiently effective, pharmacologic options may be considered. Although several medications are commonly prescribed for insomnia in the general population, particular care must be taken when selecting one for the aging adult.

The American Academy of Sleep Medicine (AASM) Clinical Practice Guideline for pharmacologic treatment of insomnia published in 2017 is used by many providers as a guide for insomnia treatment in adults.[71] Although this publication serves as a compendium of insomnia treatment data, it should be used cautiously with older adults. As the authors acknowledge, these guidelines do not contain independent analyses of efficacy in older adults and data are not stratified by age. Moreover, hypnotics are associated with an increased risk for adverse events in older adults and the starting doses listed in the guidelines do not take into account the changes in pharmacokinetics and pharmacodynamics that emerge with aging.

Many of the medications recommended by the AASM guidelines are found on the American Geriatrics Society Beers Criteria for Potentially Inappropriate Medication Use in Older Adults, which presents a list of medications to avoid in older adults when possible and is used widely by health care providers who treat this population.[72] Medications used for insomnia that are listed in the Beers Criteria include benzodiazepines, benzodiazepine receptor agonists (also known as "Z-drugs"), antihistamines, and other anticholinergic medications.

There is limited evidence for the efficacy of benzodiazepines and Z-drugs for chronic insomnia.[61] More importantly, their use can result in hangover effects, dependence, tolerance, and rebound insomnia on discontinuation. They also confer an increased risk for severe complications in older adults, including infection, depression, falls, hip fractures, car accidents, cognitive impairment, delirium, and overall mortality risk.[71,73–75]

Antihistamines, such as diphenhydramine, are sedating and unfortunately are components of many popular OTC "PM" products. Many antihistamines, particularly those used in OTC sleep aids, have anticholinergic effects such as urinary retention and constipation that are detrimental to aging adults. Anticholinergic drugs are associated with cognitive impairment and can precipitate delirium.[76,77] Antihistamines that are significantly anticholinergic should not be used in older adults.

The choice of an agent should weigh treatment goals, symptom target (sleep onset, sleep maintenance, or both), previous response to treatment, patient preference, comorbid conditions, contraindications, medication interactions, side effects, cost, and availability of other treatments.[78] Generally, medications for insomnia should be used at the lowest effective dose, dosed only intermittently rather than every night, and used in the short term—ideally for less than 1 month. When a medication is discontinued, it should be done gradually to reduce the risk of withdrawal symptoms, including rebound insomnia. Medications with shorter elimination half-lives should be favored to mitigate daytime sedation and other side effects.[13]

Food and Drug Administration (FDA)-Approved Medications for Treatment of Insomnia with Evidence Supporting Their Use in Older Adults

Orexin receptor antagonists

Suvorexant was the first dual orexin receptor antagonist (DORA) FDA-approved for the treatment of sleep-onset and sleep maintenance insomnia. It inhibits the binding of orexin A and B, both wakefulness-promoting neuropeptides, to orexin receptors. Suvorexant increases time spent in all sleep stages, preserves sleep architecture, and improves sleep maintenance, with more modest improvements in sleep onset.[79,80] Suvorexant was well tolerated over 3 months in older patients and has not been associated with significant daytime impairment such as residual sleepiness, gait instability, or memory complaints.[81] The effects of suvorexant on sleep apnea have not been well studied, so coordination with a sleep medicine specialist is advisable when there is a diagnosis or suspicion for OSA.[80]

Another DORA, lemborexant, has subsequently been FDA-approved. Comparisons between the two DORAs suggest that lemborexant may be slightly more efficacious than suvorexant but has a greater risk of daytime somnolence and higher rates of discontinuation due to adverse effects.[82]

Ramelteon

Ramelteon is a melatonin receptor agonist approved in the United States for treatment of sleep-onset and sleep maintenance insomnia. RCTs in older adults demonstrate mixed results. One meta-analysis of 13 trials with adults and older adults reported small but statistically significant improvements in subjective sleep-onset latency and subjective quality of sleep.[83] Ramelteon does not have a significant effect on sleep maintenance insomnia.[80] It does not cause central nervous system depression and is not associated with significant rebound insomnia, withdrawal effects, memory impairment, or gait instability.[80,84,85]

Doxepin

Doxepin, a tricyclic antidepressant, is the only antidepressant that is FDA-approved for insomnia, although limited to doses of 3 to 6 mg (sold as brand-name Silenor) for this indication, far less than the 75 to 150 mg typically used to treat depression. Its mechanism of action is antihistaminic; histamine is a key neurotransmitter for wakefulness.[86] At doses below 25 mg, doxepin is highly selective for H1 receptors, with minimal anticholinergic effects. The Beers Criteria notes that at doses $\leq$ 6 mg, the safety profile of doxepin is comparable to that of placebo.[72] Three RCTs in older adults using doses of 1 mg, 3 mg, and 6 mg showed efficacy for sleep maintenance insomnia with no significant hangover effects or memory impairment. Reports of the most common side effects—somnolence, nausea, and dizziness—were similar to placebo.[80] Patients with impaired renal function may have delayed clearance of doxepin, and the medication is not recommended for individuals with severe sleep apnea.[80]

Non-FDA-Approved Medications for Treatment of Insomnia

Melatonin

Endogenous melatonin production is generally reduced in aging.[61] Exogenous melatonin is sold as an OTC sleep aid, and it is used commonly due to its availability, low cost, and relatively low burden of adverse events and side effects.[87,88] Although it is approved in Europe for short-term treatment of insomnia in adults 55 years and older, it is not FDA-approved for any indication in the United States.[61] Some data suggest that it is effective for chronic insomnia, however the data are considered of "very low" quality as per the AASM Clinical Practice Guideline.[71]

A 2018 review of pharmacologic management of insomnia in older adults found that melatonin slightly improves sleep onset and duration, but these effects are limited by variability in dosing and product quality. There is little consensus on appropriate dosing of melatonin. Doses between 3 and 5 mg are typical, but some studies indicate that 0.3 to 0.5 mg can be effective, and doses of 10 mg or more are used in certain clinical situations, for example, treatment of circadian dysregulation in patients with visual impairment and treatment of RBD.[80] A 2020 review found that short-term use of melatonin was associated with improvement in sleep quality and sleep-onset latency but had an inconsistent effect on total sleep time. The authors concluded that there was inadequate evidence to confirm its efficacy for insomnia.[87] Because of its circadian phase-shifting properties (i.e., its ability to reset the timing of the internal biological clock), melatonin has a greater impact on insomnia associated with circadian misalignment such as shift work or jet lag.[89]

A limitation of currently available data is that many studies do not specify the timing of melatonin administration. When timing is noted, it can range from 15 minutes to 2 hours before bedtime. This raises an important consideration in the use of melatonin; administering melatonin when endogenous melatonin levels are already high often has minimal impact.[87,88] There is no clear consensus, but given that most preparations of melatonin take 45 to 60 minutes to become bioavailable, and perhaps longer in older adults, the drug should be administered at least an hour before the individual's typical bedtime and should be administered at the same time each night.[88]

Given the lack of high-quality evidence and variability in formulations, further research is required to establish detailed guidelines for melatonin use in older adults. However, given some evidence for its effectiveness and its relatively low risk of causing adverse events, it is worth considering before agents associated with more risk.

Trazodone

Trazodone is an antidepressant that is not FDA-approved for insomnia but is commonly prescribed by providers who treat sleep disorders in older adults, in doses typically ranging from 25 to 100 mg.[61] Its mechanism of action is via its moderate antihistamine activity. Trazodone is often seen as a preferable choice given its very low anticholinergic activity. The clinical practice guidelines from AASM suggest that its harms outweigh its benefits and recommend that clinicians do not use trazodone for sleep-onset or maintenance insomnia.[71] Salient risks in aging adults include dizziness, orthostatic hypotension, and psychomotor impairment.[90] Parkinsonism has also been reported in elderly patients taking trazodone.[91] Patients and families should be alerted of these increased risks and encouraged to monitor for side effects.

Mirtazapine

Mirtazapine is another antidepressant with an antihistaminic mechanism of action that has been shown to have some efficacy for insomnia in limited case series and open-label studies but is not FDA-approved for that use.[92] In the aging adult, mirtazapine can be a useful agent for treating insomnia with comorbid depression, particularly if poor appetite is a symptom, however it is not recommended for primary insomnia without depression, given conflicting evidence, risk of weight gain, and possible habituation to its sedative effects.[61]

OTHER NOTEWORTHY SLEEP DISORDERS IN THE AGING ADULT

It is important to recognize that insomnia in older adults can co-occur with and obfuscate the diagnosis of other sleep disorders. Moreover, patients with overlapping sleep disorders typically do not improve unless all conditions are addressed.

Obstructive Sleep Apnea

OSA is characterized by recurrent episodes of upper airway obstruction during sleep.[15] It is the most common breathing-related sleep disorder, and its frequency increases with age.[15,93] Over half of older Americans are at high risk for OSA, although most of the cases are undiagnosed.[94] Frequent underdiagnosis may be attributable to changes in clinical presentation of older adults with OSA; after the age of 60, the disease is equally as common in females as in males, obesity is not a significant risk factor, witnessed apneas and snoring are less frequently reported, and daytime sleepiness and nocturia are more common.[95,96]

OSA is associated with cognitive impairment and incidence of dementia, among many other medical and psychiatric consequences.[93,97] Importantly, treatment of this disorder with positive airway pressure is associated with lower odds of Alzheimer's dementia diagnosis, making screening, diagnosis, and treatment critical.[97] The STOP-Bang questionnaire is a useful tool for clinicians to stratify risk for OSA and triage for referral for PSG, which confirms a diagnosis.[15,60]

Rapid Eye Movement Sleep Behavior Disorder

RBD is characterized by a lack of the atonia that is normally present in REM sleep, resulting in acting out dreams with vocalizations and/or complex motor behaviors.[15] This can result in injury to the individual or to a bed partner. Most cases of RBD have an onset between ages 50 and 70.[4]

As noted in **Table 1**, RBD is associated with several medications, and treatment may begin with lowering or discontinuing offending agents if feasible. High-dose melatonin (6 to 12 mg) is the first-line treatment of RBD. Clonazepam (0.25 to 2 mg) is a commonly used second-line treatment but should be prescribed cautiously in older adults given its substantial risks and side effects.[98]

Importantly, if a patient has RBD, is not on a medication likely to cause it, and does not have another known medical condition associated with RBD, providers should consider the possibility that the patient may have or may ultimately develop a neurodegenerative disorder. There is substantial risk for an individual with idiopathic RBD to manifest Parkinson's disease or dementia with Lewy bodies in particular.[99,100] One longitudinal study of 93 patients who had idiopathic RBD and no parkinsonian or cognitive symptoms yielded an estimated 17.7% 5-year risk of developing a neurodegenerative disease. The risk was 40.6% at 10 years, and 52.4% at 12 years.[100]

Restless Leg Syndrome and Periodic Limb Movement Disorder

RLS is defined by an urge to move one's legs in response to an uncomfortable sensation in the legs that occurs at rest and is at least partially relieved by movement. The urge is worse at night (or only occurs at night), which presents a challenge for sleeping.[15] RLS worsens steadily with age until about 60 and occurs in up to 20% of adults aged 65 and older.[16,101] With late-onset RLS (after age 45), progression of symptoms is often rapid and commonly related to aggravating factors, such as medications.[102] It may share similar features with anxiety disorders, drug-induced akathisia, leg cramps, positional discomfort, tic disorders, and peripheral neuropathy, and thus a broad differential should be considered.[103] RLS may also be comorbid with any of these conditions. RLS is diagnosed based on the presence of clinical symptoms.

PLMD is characterized by repetitive contractions of the legs that occur during sleep and often overlaps with a diagnosis of RLS.[15] Up to 90% of those diagnosed with RLS demonstrate periodic leg movements in sleep.[104] PLMD is diagnosed when PSG shows more than 15 periodic limb movements per hour, and the patient reports sleep disturbance or other functional impairment.[105]

The etiologies of RLS and PLMD are uncertain, but disturbances in iron metabolism and in the central dopaminergic system are theorized to play a role.[15,103] RLS is associated with iron deficiency, with or without anemia, and ferritin levels less than 50 μg/L.[103] Iron replacement is recommended when ferritin is ≤ 75 μg/L.[106] Neither RLS nor PLMD has a poor prognosis if sleep disruption is addressed, and neither is associated with increased risk for neurodegenerative disorders.[103]

Withdrawing potentially offending medications (selective serotonin reuptake inhibitors and other antidepressants, dopamine-blocking medications, and sedating antihistamines) when feasible may improve symptoms. Bupropion is an antidepressant that may be less likely to induce or exacerbate RLS.[107]

Behavioral measures such as regular exercise and limiting alcohol and caffeine should be used and are often effective in individuals with intermittent symptoms. Alpha-2-delta ligands (such as gabapentin) have recently been recommended as the first-line pharmacologic treatment of RLS and PLMD, supplanting dopaminergic agents, which have been associated with worsening of symptoms with chronic use.[108]

Advanced Sleep–Wake Phase Disorder

ASWPD is a circadian rhythm sleep–wake disorder in which sleep quality and duration are normal but both sleep onset and wake times are "advanced" such that an individual chronically falls asleep and wakes up earlier than is desired or socially acceptable. These individuals may attempt to stay up later in the evening to maintain a "normal" sleep schedule, believing they will be able to wake up later accordingly. However, they are likely to still wake up early, given their earlier circadian phase, resulting in less total sleep time and daytime sleepiness.[15,109] A thorough sleep history and the use of a sleep diary for at least 7 days can be useful in making this diagnosis. Depression and insomnia should be excluded, as both can also cause earlier sleep onset and early morning awakening—although these conditions can be comorbid.[109]

Factors that can contribute to the development of ASWPD in older adults include altered exposure to zeitgebers (such as light, meals, activity, and social rhythms), decreased responsiveness to evening light (which would normally delay sleep), and increased responsiveness to morning bright light, which advances the internal circadian phase and makes awakening for the day more likely.[109]

The first-line treatment of ASWPD is bright light therapy in the evening.[109] There is no substantial evidence for pharmacotherapy as treatment of ASWPD. Theoretically, melatonin administration late at night or in the early morning could be used to phase delay the circadian clock, which may improve ASWPD symptoms, but there are no data to support its efficacy for this purpose.[109,110]

SUMMARY

Insomnia and other sleep disorders are prevalent in older adults and are associated with distress and negative health outcomes. A thorough sleep history and review of medical and psychiatric history, medication list, and collateral history from bed partners or caregivers are crucial to effective diagnosis and treatment planning. Non-pharmacological treatment of insomnia, particularly CBT-I, should be implemented first whenever possible. Some pharmacologic treatments for insomnia are effective but should be chosen with great caution given substantial risks for adverse events, side effects, and medication interactions.

DISCLOSURE

Drs Z.L. Cohen, P.M. Eigenberger, M.L. Conroy, and K.M. Wilkins do not have any disclosures to report. Dr K.M. Sharkey receives royalties from Wolters Kluwer for an article on Advanced Sleep-Wake Phase Disorder.

REFERENCES

1. Ancoli-Israel S, Ayalon L. Diagnosis and treatment of sleep disorders in older adults. Am J Geriatr Psychiatry 2006;14(2):95–103.
2. Ohayon MM. Epidemiology of insomnia: what we know and what we still need to learn. Sleep Med Rev 2002;6(2):97–111.
3. Vaz Fragoso CA, Gill TM. Sleep complaints in community-living older persons: a multifactorial geriatric syndrome. J Am Geriatr Soc 2007;55(11):1853–66.
4. Miner B, Kryger MH. Sleep in the aging population. Sleep Med Clin 2017; 12(1):31–8.
5. Martin MS, et al. Sleep perception in non-insomniac healthy elderly: a 3-year longitudinal study. Rejuvenation Res 2014;17(1):11–8.
6. Bethea TN, et al. Perceived racial discrimination and risk of insomnia among middle-aged and elderly Black women. Sleep 2020;43(1).
7. Ancoli-Israel S, Ayalon L, Salzman C. Sleep in the elderly: normal variations and common sleep disorders. Harv Rev Psychiatry 2008;16(5):279–86.
8. Dew MA, et al. Healthy older adults' sleep predicts all-cause mortality at 4 to 19 years of follow-up. Psychosom Med 2003;65(1):63–73.
9. Jaussent I, et al. Insomnia and daytime sleepiness are risk factors for depressive symptoms in the elderly. Sleep 2011;34(8):1103–10.
10. Yaffe K, Falvey CM, Hoang T. Connections between sleep and cognition in older adults. Lancet Neurol 2014;13(10):1017–28.
11. Palagini L, et al. Sleep loss and hypertension: a systematic review. Curr Pharm Des 2013;19(13):2409–19.
12. Laugsand LE, et al. Insomnia and the risk of acute myocardial infarction: a population study. Circulation 2011;124(19):2073–81.
13. Kamel NS, Gammack JK. Insomnia in the elderly: cause, approach, and treatment. Am J Med 2006;119(6):463–9.
14. United Nations Department of Economic and Social Affairs, Population Division. World population ageing 2020: highlights. New York, NY: United Nations; 2021.
15. A. American Psychiatric and D.S.M.T.F. American Psychiatric Association. In: Diagnostic and statistical manual of mental disorders : DSM-5. Arlington, VA: American Psychiatric Association; 2013.
16. Harrington JJ, Lee-Chiong T Jr. Sleep and older patients. Clin Chest Med 2007; 28(4):673–84.
17. Gagnon JF, et al. Rapid-eye-movement sleep behaviour disorder and neurodegenerative diseases. Lancet Neurol 2006;5(5):424–32.
18. Thompson C, et al. A portrait of obstructive sleep apnea risk factors in 27,210 middle-aged and older adults in the Canadian Longitudinal Study on Aging. Sci Rep 2022;12(1):5127.

19. Ohayon MM, et al. Meta-analysis of quantitative sleep parameters from childhood to old age in healthy individuals: developing normative sleep values across the human lifespan. Sleep 2004;27(7):1255–73.

20. Institute of Medicine Committee on Sleep, M. and Research. In: Colten HR, Altevogt BM, editors. The national academies collection: reports funded by national institutes of health, in Sleep Disorders and Sleep Deprivation: an Unmet Public Health Problem. Washington (DC): National Academies Press (US)Copyright © 2006, National Academy of Sciences; 2006.

21. S., I.C.A.-I., C. A., et al. The AASM manual for the scoring of sleep and associated events: rules, terminology, and technical specification. Westchester, IL: American Academy of Sleep Medicine; 2007.

22. Moser D, et al. Sleep classification according to AASM and Rechtschaffen & Kales: effects on sleep scoring parameters. Sleep 2009;32(2):139–49.

23. Carskadon MA, Dement WC. Chapter 2 - normal human sleep: an overview. In: Kryger M, Roth T, Dement WC, editors. Principles and practice of sleep medicine. 6th edition. Philadelphia, PA: Elsevier; 2017. p. 15–24.e3.

24. Siegel JM. The REM sleep-memory consolidation hypothesis. Science 2001; 294(5544):1058–63.

25. Hirshkowitz M, et al. National Sleep Foundation's sleep time duration recommendations: methodology and results summary. Sleep Health 2015;1(1):40–3.

26. Ensrud KE, et al. Sleep Disturbances and Frailty Status in Older Community-Dwelling Men. J Am Geriatr Soc 2009;57(11):2085–93.

27. Min Y, Slattum PW. Poor sleep and risk of falls in community-dwelling older adults: a systematic review. J Appl Gerontol 2018;37(9):1059–84.

28. Neikrug AB, Ancoli-Israel S. Sleep disorders in the older adult - a mini-review. Gerontology 2010;56(2):181–9.

29. Duffy JF, et al. Peak of circadian melatonin rhythm occurs later within the sleep of older subjects. Am J Physiol Endocrinol Metab 2002;282(2):E297–303.

30. Monk TH. Aging human circadian rhythms: conventional wisdom may not always be right. J Biol Rhythms 2005;20(4):366–74.

31. Burgess HJ, et al. The Relationship Between the Dim Light Melatonin Onset and Sleep on a Regular Schedule in Young Healthy Adults. Behav Sleep Med 2003; 1(2):102–14.

32. Woodward M. Insomnia in the elderly. Aust Fam Physician 1999;28(7):653–8.

33. Klerman EB, et al. Older people awaken more frequently but fall back asleep at the same rate as younger people. Sleep 2004;27(4):793–8.

34. Kocevska D, et al. Sleep characteristics across the lifespan in 1.1 million people from the Netherlands, United Kingdom and United States: a systematic review and meta-analysis. Nat Hum Behav 2021;5(1):113–22.

35. Vitiello MV, Moe KE, Prinz PN. Sleep complaints cosegregate with illness in older adults: Clinical research informed by and informing epidemiological studies of sleep. J Psychosom Res 2002;53(1):555–9.

36. Glidewell RN, Moorcroft WH, Lee-Chiong T. Comorbid Insomnia: Reciprocal Relationships and Medication Management. Sleep Med Clin 2010;5(4):627–46.

37. Foley D, et al. Sleep disturbances and chronic disease in older adults: results of the 2003 National Sleep Foundation Sleep in America Survey. J Psychosom Res 2004;56(5):497–502.

38. Taylor DJ, et al. Comorbidity of Chronic Insomnia With Medical Problems. Sleep 2007;30(2):213–8.

39. Dragioti E, et al. Association of insomnia severity with well-being, quality of life and health care costs: A cross-sectional study in older adults with chronic pain (PainS65+). Eur J Pain 2018;22(2):414–25.

40. Mander BA, et al. Sleep: a novel mechanistic pathway, biomarker, and treatment target in the pathology of Alzheimer's disease? Trends Neurosci 2016;39(8): 552–66.

41. Walsh JK, et al. Nighttime Insomnia Symptoms and Perceived Health in the America Insomnia Survey (AIS). Sleep 2011;34(8):997–1011.

42. Wastesson JW, et al. An update on the clinical consequences of polypharmacy in older adults: a narrative review. Expert Opin Drug Saf 2018;17(12):1185–96.

43. Barczi SR, Teodorescu MC. Psychiatric and medical comorbidities and effects of medications in older adults. In: Principles and practice of sleep medicine. Philadelphia, PA: Elsevier, Inc.; 2022. p. 1795–806.e6. Chapter 191.

44. Whittom S, et al. Effects of melatonin and bright light administration on motor and sensory symptoms of RLS. Sleep Med 2010;11(4):351–5.

45. Shinno H. Effect of levothyroxine on prolonged nocturnal sleep time and excessive daytime somnolence in patients with idiopathic hypersomnia. Sleep Med 2011;12(6):578–83.

46. Van Gastel A. Drug-Induced Insomnia and Excessive Sleepiness. Sleep Med Clin 2018;13(2):147–59.

47. Zimmerman ME, et al. Are sleep onset/maintenance difficulties associated with medical or psychiatric comorbidities in nondemented community-dwelling older adults? J Clin Sleep Med 2013;9(4):363–9.

48. Komulainen K, et al. Association of depressive symptoms with health care utilization in older adults: Longitudinal evidence from the Survey of Health, Aging, and Retirement in Europe. Int J Geriatr Psychiatry 2021;36(4):521–9.

49. Dew MA, et al. Temporal profiles of the course of depression during treatment. Predictors of pathways toward recovery in the elderly. Arch Gen Psychiatry 1997;54(11):1016–24.

50. Gallo JJ, et al. Role of persistent and worsening sleep disturbance in depression remission and suicidal ideation among older primary care patients: the PROSPECT study. Sleep 2020;43(10).

51. Ohayon MM, Shapiro CM. Sleep disturbances and psychiatric disorders associated with posttraumatic stress disorder in the general population. Compr Psychiatry 2000;41(6):469–78.

52. Jackson A, Cavanagh J, Scott J. A systematic review of manic and depressive prodromes. J Affect Disord 2003;74(3):209–17.

53. Chang A-M, et al. Evening use of light-emitting eReaders negatively affects sleep, circadian timing, and next-morning alertness. Proc Natl Acad Sci 2015; 112(4):1232–7.

54. Lancel M, Stroebe M, Eisma MC. Sleep disturbances in bereavement: a systematic review. Sleep Med Rev 2020;53:101331.

55. Ong JC, Arendt T, Kalmbach D, et al. Insomnia Diagnosis, Assessment, and Evaluation. In: Principles and practice of sleep medicine. Elsevier, Inc.; 2022. p. 858–66.e2.

56. Lichstein KL, et al. Quantitative criteria for insomnia. Behav Res Ther 2003; 41(4):427–45.

57. Carney CE, et al. The consensus sleep diary: standardizing prospective sleep self-monitoring. Sleep 2012;35(2):287–302.

58. Morin CM, et al. The Insomnia Severity Index: psychometric indicators to detect insomnia cases and evaluate treatment response. Sleep 2011;34(5):601–8.

59. Buysse DJ, et al. The Pittsburgh Sleep Quality Index: a new instrument for psychiatric practice and research. Psychiatry Res 1989;28(2):193–213.

60. Chung F, Abdullah HR, Liao P. STOP-Bang Questionnaire: A Practical Approach to Screen for Obstructive Sleep Apnea. Chest 2016;149(3):631–8.

61. Patel D, Steinberg J, Patel P. Insomnia in the Elderly: A Review. J Clin Sleep Med 2018;14(6):1017–24.

62. Morin CM, et al. Behavioral and pharmacological therapies for late-life insomnia: a randomized controlled trial. JAMA 1999;281(11):991–9.

63. Geiger-Brown JM, et al. Cognitive behavioral therapy in persons with comorbid insomnia: A meta-analysis. Sleep Med Rev 2015;23:54–67.

64. Irwin MR, Cole JC, Nicassio PM. Comparative meta-analysis of behavioral interventions for insomnia and their efficacy in middle-aged adults and in older adults 55+ years of age. Health Psychol 2006;25(1):3–14.

65. Perini F, et al. Mindfulness-based therapy for insomnia for older adults with sleep difficulties: a randomized clinical trial. Psychol Med 2021;1:1–11.

66. Carney CE, Danforth M. Behavioral Treatment I: Therapeutic Approaches and Implementation. In: Principles and practice of sleep medicine. Philadelphia, PA: Elsevier, Inc.; 2022. p. 883–9.e4.

67. Reidel BW. Sleep hygiene. In: Lichstein KLM, C.M., editors. Treatment of late life insomnia. Thousand Oaks, CA: Sage Publications, Inc; 2000. p. 125–46.

68. Qaseem A, et al. Management of Chronic Insomnia Disorder in Adults: A Clinical Practice Guideline From the American College of Physicians. Ann Intern Med 2016;165(2):125–33.

69. Manber R, et al. CBT for insomnia in patients with high and low depressive symptom severity: adherence and clinical outcomes. J Clin Sleep Med 2011; 7(6):645–52.

70. Cheng P, et al. Efficacy of digital CBT for insomnia to reduce depression across demographic groups: a randomized trial. Psychol Med 2019;49(3):491–500.

71. Sateia MJ, et al. Clinical Practice Guideline for the Pharmacologic Treatment of Chronic Insomnia in Adults: An American Academy of Sleep Medicine Clinical Practice Guideline. J Clin Sleep Med 2017;13(2):307–49.

72. By the american geriatrics society beers criteria update expert, P American geriatrics society 2019 updated AGS beers criteria(R) for potentially inappropriate medication use in older adults. J Am Geriatr Soc 2019;67(4):674–94.

73. Crowe SF, Stranks EK. The residual medium and long-term cognitive effects of benzodiazepine use: an updated meta-analysis. Arch Clin Neuropsychol 2018; 33(7):901–11.

74. Donnelly K, et al. Benzodiazepines, Z-drugs and the risk of hip fracture: A systematic review and meta-analysis. PLoS One 2017;12(4):e0174730.

75. Inouye SK. Delirium in older persons. N Engl J Med 2006;354(11):1157–65.

76. Egberts A, et al. Anticholinergic drug burden and delirium: a systematic review. J Am Med Dir Assoc 2021;22(1):65–73.e4.

77. Ruxton K, Woodman RJ, Mangoni AA. Drugs with anticholinergic effects and cognitive impairment, falls and all-cause mortality in older adults: A systematic review and meta-analysis. Br J Clin Pharmacol 2015;80(2):209–20.

78. Schutte-Rodin S, et al. Clinical guideline for the evaluation and management of chronic insomnia in adults. J Clin Sleep Med 2008;4(5):487–504.

79. Snyder E, et al. Effects of suvorexant on sleep architecture and power spectral profile in patients with insomnia: analysis of pooled phase 3 data. Sleep Med 2016;19:93–100.

80. Abad VC, Guilleminault C. Insomnia in Elderly Patients: Recommendations for Pharmacological Management. Drugs Aging 2018;35(9):791–817.
81. Herring WJ, et al. Suvorexant in elderly patients with insomnia: pooled analyses of data from phase iii randomized controlled clinical trials. Am J Geriatr Psychiatry 2017;25(7):791–802.
82. Kishi T. Lemborexant vs suvorexant for insomnia: a systematic review and network meta-analysis. J Psychiatr Res 2020;128:68–74.
83. Kuriyama A, Honda M, Hayashino Y. Ramelteon for the treatment of insomnia in adults: a systematic review and meta-analysis. Sleep Med 2014;15(4):385–92.
84. Zammit G, et al. Effect of ramelteon on middle-of-the-night balance in older adults with chronic insomnia. J Clin Sleep Med 2009;5(1):34–40.
85. Roth T, et al. Effects of ramelteon on patient-reported sleep latency in older adults with chronic insomnia. Sleep Med 2006;7(4):312–8.
86. Rojas-Fernandez CH, Chen Y. Use of ultra-low-dose (≤6 mg) doxepin for treatment of insomnia in older people. Can Pharm J (Ott) 2014;147(5):281–9.
87. Low TL, Choo FN, Tan SM. The efficacy of melatonin and melatonin agonists in insomnia - an umbrella review. J Psychiatr Res 2020;121:10–23.
88. Cipolla-Neto J, Amaral FGD. Melatonin as a hormone: new physiological and clinical insights. Endocr Rev 2018;39(6):990–1028.
89. Sharkey KM, Eastman CI. Melatonin phase shifts human circadian rhythms in a placebo-controlled simulated night-work study. Am J Physiol Regul Integr Comp Physiol 2002;282(2):R454–63.
90. Mendelson WB. A review of the evidence for the efficacy and safety of trazodone in insomnia. J Clin Psychiatry 2005;66(4):469–76.
91. Sarwar AI. Trazodone and Parkinsonism: The Link Strengthens. Clin Neuropharmacol 2018;41(3):106–8.
92. Atkin T, Comai S, Gobbi G. Drugs for Insomnia beyond Benzodiazepines: Pharmacology, Clinical Applications, and Discovery. Pharmacol Rev 2018;70(2):197–245.
93. Russell T, Duntley S. Sleep disordered breathing in the elderly. Am J Med 2011;124(12):1123–6.
94. Braley TJ, et al. Recognition and diagnosis of obstructive sleep apnea in older Americans. J Am Geriatr Soc 2018;66(7):1296–302.
95. Phillips B. Obstructive sleep apnea in older adults. In: Kryger MH, Roth T, Dement WC, editors. Principles and practice of sleep medicine. Philadelphia, PA: Elsevier; 2022.
96. Endeshaw Y. Clinical characteristics of obstructive sleep apnea in community-dwelling older adults. J Am Geriatr Soc 2006;54(11):1740–4.
97. Dunietz GL, et al. Obstructive sleep apnea treatment and dementia risk in older adults. Sleep 2021;44(9).
98. Jung Y, St Louis EK. Treatment of REM Sleep Behavior Disorder. Curr Treat Options Neurol 2016;18(11):50.
99. Boeve BF. REM sleep behavior disorder: updated review of the core features, the REM sleep behavior disorder-neurodegenerative disease association, evolving concepts, controversies, and future directions. Ann N Y Acad Sci 2010;1184:15–54.
100. Postuma RB, et al. Quantifying the risk of neurodegenerative disease in idiopathic REM sleep behavior disorder. Neurology 2009;72(15):1296–300.
101. Ohayon MM, O'Hara R, Vitiello MV. Epidemiology of restless legs syndrome: a synthesis of the literature. Sleep Med Rev 2012;16(4):283–95.

102. Allen RP, Earley CJ. Defining the phenotype of the restless legs syndrome (RLS) using age-of-symptom-onset. Sleep Med 2000;1(1):11–9.
103. Hategan A, et al. Geriatric psychiatry: a case-based textbook. Springer International Publishing; 2018.
104. Trotti LM, et al. Correlates of PLMs variability over multiple nights and impact upon RLS diagnosis. Sleep Med 2009;10(6):668–71.
105. Sateia MJ. International classification of sleep disorders-Third Edition. Chest 2014;146(5):1387–94.
106. Allen RP, et al. Evidence-based and consensus clinical practice guidelines for the iron treatment of restless legs syndrome/Willis-Ekbom disease in adults and children: an IRLSSG task force report. Sleep Med 2018;41:27–44.
107. Natter J, Yokoyama T, Michel B. Relative frequency of drug-induced sleep disorders for 32 antidepressants in a large set of Internet user reviews. Sleep 2021; 44(12).
108. Silber MH, et al. The management of restless legs syndrome: an updated algorithm. Mayo Clin Proc 2021;96(7):1921–37.
109. Sharkey K. Advanced sleep-wake phase disorder. In: Eichler A, editor. UpToDate. Waltham (MA): UpToDate; 2022. Accessed on April 10, 2022.
110. Sack RL, et al. Circadian rhythm sleep disorders: part II, advanced sleep phase disorder, delayed sleep phase disorder, free-running disorder, and irregular sleep-wake rhythm. An American Academy of Sleep Medicine review. Sleep 2007;30(11):1484–501.

Psychopharmacology in the Elderly: Why Does Age Matter?

Kripa Balaram, MD[a], Silpa Balachandran, MD[b],*

KEYWORDS

- Psychopharmacology • Elderly • Psychotropics • Antipsychotics • Antidepressants
- Sedative-hypnotics • Metabolism • Mood stabilizers

KEY POINTS

- Older adults are more likely to have several underlying medical illnesses, leading to an increased risk of polypharmacy and its associated drug-drug interactions.
- Generally, physiological changes due to aging affect most of the pharmacokinetic processes in the body.
- Age-related physiologic changes in cardiovascular, gastric, hepatic, and renal function can lead to changes in the pharmacokinetics of medications that can affect the absorption, distribution, accumulation, and clearance and elimination of various medications.
- Age-related physiologic changes further increase sensitivity of serious and potentially fatal adverse reactions such as orthostatic hypotension, cognitive impairment, arrhythmias, falls, delirium, and death.
- Current clinical trials rarely include older adults. Therefore, there is an ever-increasing need for continued research into the efficacy and safety of pharmacotherapy options for use in this population.

INTRODUCTION

According to census data, there are more than 45 million adults older than 65 years living in the United States. This number is projected to reach 64 million by 2030 and 90 million by 2050.[1] This growing percentage of the population also represents an increasing number of individuals who meet criteria for neuropsychiatric disorders. Estimates from the CDC indicate that anywhere from 1% to 5% of older adults meet criteria for major depressive disorder.[2] These estimates are vastly increased in those with medical comorbidities or physical limitations, particularly those requiring intensive home care or hospitalization.[2] More than 5% of those between age 65 and 75

[a] Department of Psychiatry, MetroHealth Medical Center, Case Western Reserve University School of Medicine, 2500 MetroHealth Drive, Cleveland, OH 44109, USA; [b] Northeast Ohio Medical University, Adult and Geriatric Psychiatry, Akron general-Cleveland Clinic, 1 Akron General Avenue, Akron, OH, 44307, USA
* Corresponding author.
E-mail address: Balachs2@ccf.org

Psychiatr Clin N Am 45 (2022) 735–744
https://doi.org/10.1016/j.psc.2022.07.004
0193-953X/22/© 2022 Elsevier Inc. All rights reserved.
psych.theclinics.com

years and up to 35% of those older than 85 years meet criteria for a major neurocognitive disorder, especially for Alzheimer dementia.[3] Although rates vary greatly based on the type of dementia and several underlying psychosocial factors, anywhere from 30% to 50% of individuals experience agitation, psychosis, or other behavioral disturbances. These neuropsychiatric changes often require some level of pharmacologic intervention for management.[4] Some estimates indicate that psychotropics are the most frequently prescribed among all medication classes in this particular population.[5] Given this growing percentage of the population that is aging and the significant subset within that population that require psychotropic medications for management of various neuropsychiatric conditions, there is an increasing need for clinicians to become familiar with the unique challenges and considerations that apply when prescribing medications.

Generally, aging affects most of the pharmacokinetic processes in the body.[4–17] These age-related changes can be observed in all the pharmacological mechanisms that are involved in drug distribution, absorption, metabolism, and clearance.[5] Older adults are more likely to have underlying medical illnesses, several preexisting comorbidities, and overall declining health. Because of this, older adults are more likely to be prescribed a greater number of medications at one time,[5] which leads to potentially dangerous drug-drug interactions that can lead to alterations in the active concentrations of individual medications. These drug-drug interactions can ultimately increase risk of delirium or cognitive impairment, enhance the risk of potentially dangerous adverse effects, and increase overall risk of mortality.[5]

These unique risks and challenges underline the inclusion of most psychotropic medications, including tricyclic antidepressants, benzodiazepines, some antiepileptic mood stabilizers, and some antipsychotics, within the Beer's Criteria for Potentially Inappropriate Medication Use in Older Adults.[6] Clinicians must therefore be comfortable with managing these individuals in the context of their entire health status, including medical comorbidities and complicated medication regimens. Clinicians must also remain familiar with the special considerations that are present when prescribing psychotropic medications in the elderly (Table 1).

SPECIAL CONSIDERATIONS IN PRESCRIBING PSYCHOTROPIC MEDICATIONS IN THE ELDERLY

The inclusion criteria of most clinical trials generally favor the enrollment of younger, healthier participants with fewer medical or psychiatric comorbidities to reduce the risk of confounding factors,[7,8] whichleads to the exclusion of older adults from trials, in particular those that assess the safety and efficacy of newly developed medications; this has led to an overall lack of evidence supporting or discouraging the use of various medications within the geriatric population.

Older adults are more likely to have several underlying medical illnesses, particularly those of a neurovascular or cardiovascular nature.[2] Because of this, they are more likely to be prescribed a greater number of medications at one time, often with some unintentional overlap between pharmacological effects.[9] This potential polypharmacy leads directly to an increased risk of associated drug-drug interactions, which can alter the metabolism of each medication that is administered, lead to the accumulation of toxic metabolites, and increase the risk of side effects and adverse reactions.[10,11] Some estimates indicate that the risk of adverse drug reactions increases exponentially with every new medication that is added.[5,9] Because of the effects of polypharmacy on the pathways of medication metabolism, particularly absorption and clearance, serum concentrations of medications can oftentimes be

Table 1
Common age-related pharmacokinetic changes[10,15]

Physiologic Characteristic	Age-Related Changes	Possible Associated Adverse Effect
Absorption	• Decreased hydrochloric acid secretion, increased gastric pH • Decreased gastric motility and emptying	• Most psychotropics are not affected • Can lead to drug-drug interactions between medications that can further slow gastric motility
Serum Concentration	• Decrease of lean muscle mass and total body water and increase in total fat content • Leads to an increased volume of distribution of medications	• Prolonged elimination of lipophilic medications • Increased accumulation of medication • Most psychotropic medications, except lithium, will accumulate in the body
Renal function	• Decreased renal blood flow • Decreased glomerular filtration rate • Decreased creatinine production • Decreased clearance capacity due to tubular dysfunction	• Decreased clearance of some medications, particularly lithium • Accumulation of metabolites, particularly for antidepressants • Metabolites can be cardiotoxic
Hepatic function	• Decreased hepatic blood flow • Decreased total hepatic mass • Decreased hepatic enzyme activity	• Increased concentrations of unmetabolized medications leads to accumulation • Decreased clearance of most psychotropic medications

Normal aging processes can lead to several changes in the metabolism of medications. This, in turn, can lead to possible adverse effects. This table provides a general overview of the age-related changes that can be observed in the pharmacokinetics of drug metabolism.

greater or less than clinically indicated or physiologically tolerated[9]; this can further lead to difficulties in dose titration in a population that is already susceptible to adverse reactions and side effects.

Aging-related changes in drug metabolism may lead to changes in the absorption, total maximum concentration, time to reach maximum concentration, volume of distribution of the medication, or the rates of elimination of medications.[8,9] Similar to the risks of polypharmacy, this can lead to increased or decreased bioavailability due to medication doses that are unintentionally subtherapeutic or supratherapeutic.[12] These metabolic changes can also cause medications, once in the body, to elicit more potent therapeutic responses.[12]

In addition, changes in medication metabolism due to the processes of normal physiologic aging can lead to an increased risk of dependency with the use of medications with abuse potential, such as benzodiazepines, barbiturates, or stimulants, and cause more severe symptoms of withdrawal upon discontinuation.[12] Furthermore, in the elderly, any possible signs of medication dependence or substance use—such as confusion and cognitive impairment, personality changes, or falls—can also be confused with the general physiological changes associated with aging or with other organic neurodegenerative processes.[12]

Commonly occurring disease states in older adults can also contribute to an increased risk of adverse effects when psychotropic medications are prescribed.

Some examples of this include an increase in the risk of sexual dysfunction in those with preexisting atherosclerosis, an increase in the risk of anticholinergic-induced urinary retention and renal dysfunction in those with preexisting bladder outlet obstruction, and an increase in the risk of constipation and small bowel obstruction that can be exacerbated with the use of anticholinergic or neuroleptic medications in those with preexisting bowel hypomotility.[13]

PHARMACOLOGICAL CONSIDERATIONS IN PRESCRIBING PSYCHOTROPIC MEDICATIONS IN THE ELDERLY

There are several physiologic changes that occur in the context of normal aging that can lead to differences in the therapeutic effects of medications when administered in the elderly.

The skin undergoes several structural and functional changes with aging. When coupled with overall reduced tissue perfusion, this can affect the absorption and subsequent bioavailability of medications that are administered transdermally.[8] For example, the acetylcholinesterase inhibitor rivastigmine, the monoamine oxidase inhibitor selegiline, and lidocaine have been formulated as transdermal patches, generally to achieve consistent 24-hour dosing or to circumvent any possible gastrointestinal side effects.[14] Disruptions in skin integrity and reduced tissue blood perfusion can lead to decreased absorption of these medications with subsequent concentrations in the body that are subtherapeutic and, potentially, ineffective.

Several physiologic changes also take place in the gastrointestinal system with age. These changes include a decrease in hydrochloric acid and pepsin secretion, an increase in gastric emptying times, a decrease in gastric motility, an increase in baseline gastric pH, and an overall decrease in gastric and intestinal blood flow.[7,8,10] These changes can lead to alterations in the bioavailability of enteric-coated or pH-dependent medications. In addition, reduced gastric blood flow, decreased gastric acid secretion, and impaired gastric motility can also affect medication absorption.[7,8]

Other age-related changes include a decrease in total body muscle mass, an increase in total body water, and an increase in total body fat percentage; this leads to increased serum concentrations of hydrophilic medications, such as some of the beta blocking agents, and decreased serum concentrations of lipophilic medications, such as the benzodiazepine diazepam. In addition, lipophilic medications take longer to reach steady state due to the higher concentrations of total body water.[8] They may also accumulate with repeated dosing.[8] Because of an overall decrease in serum albumin concentrations and an increase in alpha1-acid glycoprotein with age, protein binding ability decreases, which causes alterations in the metabolism of medications that are highly protein-bound, such as diazepam or phenytoin.[10,15]

Over time, renal function can be impaired by a steady age-related decline in renal blood flow and glomerular filtration rates. There are also noted decreases in creatinine production and overall clearance capacity due to tubular dysfunction. Impaired renal function can also be caused by other underlying medical conditions, such as hypertension or diabetes. In clinical practice, this usually translates to a need for dose adjustments in those with known renal impairment or dysfunction.[8] Lithium is a well-known example of a medication that must be used cautiously in those with renal impairment.[8]

Similarly, hepatic function is affected by reduced hepatic blood flow, reduced total liver mass, and a decline in the function of the hepatic enzyme pathway systems[8]; this, in turn, leads to a significant increase in the serum concentrations and bioavailability of medications that undergo extensive first-pass metabolism for deactivation, elimination, and clearance. Examples of psychotropic medications that can be affected by these changes include amitriptyline, lidocaine, and propranolol.[8] Alternatively, there will be a marked decrease in the serum concentrations and the bioavailability of medications that require activation through various hepatic enzymatic pathways.[8] This, in turn, can result in an increase in the time required for a medication to reach therapeutic concentrations and can also lead to an increase in the rates of accumulation and time for clearance once these concentrations are achieved.[5] Other notable changes due to declining hepatic function include an increased concentration of partially metabolized or unmetabolized medications that require activation through first pass metabolism and prolonged exposures to medications that require deactivation through hepatic enzyme pathways before elimination.[5] These accumulating medications or metabolites are often toxic to various organ systems, in particular the cardiovascular and central nervous system, and can contribute to the extensive side-effect profiles that are often observed in this particular population.[5,8]

In the elderly, both the number of dopaminergic neurons and dopamine receptors are significantly decreased,[8,10] which can lead to a number of the commonly observed adverse reactions and side effects observed in this population, particularly those seen with the administration of neuroleptic agents. The most commonly observed side effects in this population, therefore, include the risks of developing delirium or tardive dyskinesias, both of which are mediated by dopamine blockade or receptor hypersensitivity.[8,10] Ultimately, this increased dopaminergic sensitivity is also the proposed mechanism behind the overall increase in risk of mortality from use of any neuroleptics.[8,10]

An overall age-related physiologic decline in cognitive function, along with increased permeability of the blood-brain barrier, can lead to increased concentrations of medications in the central nervous system,[8] and this leads to an associated increase in the therapeutic responses to these medications.[8] Both alpha and beta noradrenergic receptor quantities and receptor responsiveness are also decreased with age, leading to a decrease in the effectiveness in the elderly of commonly used psychotropic medications, such as clonidine or propranolol.[10] Normal physiological aging processes also lead to a loss in cholinergic neurons and decreased function of choline acetyltransferase, the enzyme involved in acetylcholine synthesis.[10] These changes contribute to a susceptibility for the development of delirium and to the possibility of anticholinergic toxicity in this population.[10,16] The regulatory mechanisms that maintain physiological homeostasis are also somewhat impaired with age, causing older adults to be more susceptible to some generalized side effects, such as hypotension[8] (Table 2).

CONSIDERATIONS WHEN PRESCRIBING SPECIFIC MEDICATION CLASSES IN THE ELDERLY
Antidepressants

Tricyclic antidepressants used to be the mainstay of the treatment of depression in all adults, including the elderly. However, this medication class has largely fallen out of favor due to numerous potentially dangerous side effects, including cardiovascular dysfunction, falls, electrolyte disturbances, and anticholinergic toxicity exacerbated by the accumulation of toxic metabolites.[13,17] These anticholinergic effects, which include dry mouth, blurred vision, and urinary retention, can be particularly bothersome in the elderly due to underlying medical comorbidities.[7] Older adults are, in general, more likely to experience these adverse effects with tricyclic antidepressant use due to both underlying medical conditions and the general pharmacokinetic and pharmacodynamic changes associated with aging.

Table 2
Common age-related adverse effects of psychotropics in the elderly[17]

Medication	Common Use or Indication	Adverse Effects
Tricyclic antidepressants	Depression	• Delayed metabolism causes accumulation of metabolites • More sensitivity to anticholinergic side effects: dry mouth, constipation, urinary retention, delirium • Can be too sedating or too activating for some • More sensitive to noradrenergic side effects: orthostatic hypotension • More sensitive to cardiac side effects: arrhythmias, conduction disturbances
Lithium	Bipolar disorder	• Half-life and serum levels are increased and prolonged • Clearance and elimination are slowed • Antihypertensives commonly use in the elderly can lead to potentially fatal drug-drug interactions
Monoamine oxidase inhibitors	Depression	• Orthostatic hypotension • Difficulty with dietary restrictions • Can be too sedating or too activating for some • Risk of hypertensive crisis
Antipsychotics	Psychosis, agitation, mood stabilization	• Increased sensitivity to extrapyramidal symptoms • Increased occurrence of tardive dyskinesia • Increased risk of orthostatic hypotension • Increased risk of anticholinergic toxicity
Benzodiazepines	Anxiety, agitation, disruptive behavior in the elderly	• Increased sensitivity to sedative effects • Risk of disinhibition paradoxical activation and agitation • Risk of memory impairment and cognitive blunting • Risk of falls • Prolonged half-life and decreased clearance of protein-bound benzodiazepines such as diazepam, chlordiazepoxides, and oxazepam • Risk of accumulation of longer-acting benzodiazepines

The psychotropic medications that are commonly prescribed in the elderly are often affected by normal physiological processes associated with aging. This table provides a basic outline of some of the adverse effects that can occur in the elderly, due to these age-related changes, when prescribing these psychotropic medications.

Monoamine oxidase inhibitors are another class of antidepressant medications that have fallen out of favor in recent times, mainly due to the necessity of a potentially restrictive tyramine-free diet and the risks of hypotension and falls.[13] However, when compared with tricyclic antidepressants, monoamine oxidase inhibitors have relatively low risks of anticholinergic or antihistaminergic side effects along with little to no observed effects of cardiovascular or neurocognitive function.[13]

Selective serotonin reuptake inhibitors, or SSRIs, are generally considered to be the first-line treatment of depression in all adults, including the elderly. Studies have not proved one selective serotonin reuptake inhibitor to be superior over another in terms of efficacy or side-effect profile, and they are generally considered to be better tolerated among the currently available antidepressant classes due to fewer anticholinergic, cardiovascular, and neurocognitive side effects.[18] The exception is paroxetine, which has similar side effects to nortriptyline. However, side effects present across the medication class—such as hyponatremia, appetite disturbances and weight loss, and sexual dysfunction—occur more frequently and at lower medication doses in older adults.[18] Additional care must also be taken when combining multiple antidepressants due to drug-drug interactions and an exponentially increased risk of serotonin syndrome.[7]

Antipsychotics

Antipsychotic medications can be used for a number of indications in the elderly including psychosis due to both an organic psychiatric disorder or an underlying medical or neurocognitive disorder, mood disturbances, or agitation associated with delirium or dementia.[19] Two antipsychotic medications, clozapine and pimavanserin, have also received Food and Drug Administration approval for the use of Parkinson disease psychosis. Although these medications have become widespread in their use in older adults, their use carries a unique set of risks in this population. The United States Food and Drug Administration has issued a black box warning identifying an overall increased risk of mortality with the use of antipsychotic medications in older adults.[20]

Antipsychotics, across their medication class, have a risk of anticholinergic and adrenergic side effects. These side effects, which include constipation, urinary retention, delirium, or orthostatic hypotension and associated risk of falls, are more likely to occur in the elderly due to the pharmacodynamic changes associated with aging.[17,19] Atypical antipsychotic medications, such as quetiapine or olanzapine, are more likely to cause metabolic disturbances. These disturbances, which can include dyslipidemias and hyperglycemia, can exacerbate and further complicate the management of underlying metabolic or cardiovascular conditions that are often present in this population.[19] Because of decreased dopaminergic production and receptor activity, older adults are also at increased risk of developing extrapyramidal symptoms and tardive dyskinesias with antipsychotic use.[17]

Mood Stabilizers

The use of Lithium in older adults for mood stabilization requires special considerations due to the risk of impaired medication metabolism caused by underlying renal dysfunction.[17] This results in increased risk of supratherapeutic levels, and associated toxicity creates a need for more frequent monitoring of serum Lithium levels along with regular monitoring of renal and thyroid function.[17] The drug-drug interactions caused by common antihypertensive medications, which are almost universally used in this particular population, can also lead to sub- or supratherapeutic medication levels.[17]

Valproic acid is currently used for both mood stabilization and for the agitated and disinhibited behavior that can be seen in delirium or dementia.[21] Because of the reduced hepatic function that is often seen in this age group and the increased risk of drug-drug interactions, frequent monitoring of serum valproic acid levels is essential, along with regular assessments of both serum platelet counts and hepatic function.[21] The most common side effects with valproic acid use, including gastrointestinal distress, sedation, ataxia, and hepatotoxicity, occur more frequently and at lower doses in older adults.[7]

Cholinesterase Inhibitors

Cholinesterase inhibitors, such as rivastigmine and donepezil, are commonly used in the management of neurocognitive disorders in the elderly. There have also been some reports of these medications having neuroprotective and cardioprotective effects in older adults.[22] In general, cholinesterase inhibitors are considered to be safe for use in this population. However, the presence of other medications with anticholinergic properties, such as antipsychotics or antihistaminergic agents, can cause drug-drug interactions that could lead to potentially dangerous side effects as well as antagonism of different medication effects.[23]

Sedative-Hypnotics

Benzodiazepines pose a unique set of challenges when used in the elderly. Pharmacologically, the slowed metabolism and decreased clearance of some benzodiazepines, particularly those that are longer-acting, can lead to the accumulation of both the medications and their metabolites.[17] Older adults are also more sensitive to the sedative effects of benzodiazepines, along with increased risk of falls, cognitive blunting, cerebellar dysfunction, and memory impairment.[7,17] There is also some observed risk of a paradoxical disinhibition or agitated activation that can be observed with the use of benzodiazepines in the elderly.[17]

Barbiturates were previously prescribed with greater frequency for anxiety and insomnia in the elderly. However, these have largely fallen out of favor due to potentially dangerous side effects, including sedation, disorientation and confusion, paradoxical agitation, and risk of dependence and withdrawal.[7]

Zolpidem, a nonbenzodiazepine hypnotic, was previously favored over benzodiazepines for use in older adults. However, recent data have indicated an increased risk of falls with associated risk of fractures, cognitive impairment, and accumulation of metabolites.[24] Other, newer nonbenzodiazepine hypnotics such as suvorexant are generally well tolerated but there are limited safety data from which statistically significant conclusions can be drawn.

SUMMARY

In general, prescribing psychotropic medications in the geriatric population comes with a unique set of considerations and challenges. The normal physiological changes associated with aging contribute to alterations in the pharmacodynamic and pharmacokinetic processes in which medications are metabolized within the body. These age-related changes can lead to changes in the absorption, enzymatic activation, serum concentration and bioavailability, and clearance and elimination of medications; this can, in turn, lead to the unintentional accumulation of medications or their metabolites within the body or to levels of medications that are persistently sub- or supratherapeutic. These factors all ultimately contribute to the development of adverse effects.

These pharmacodynamic and pharmacokinetic changes in medication metabolism are further complicated by the possibility of several underlying medical and neuropsychiatric comorbidities in this population with an associated overall decline in health; this also contributes to the very legitimate risks caused by polypharmacy and any resulting drug-drug interactions.

These challenges can be prevented or, at the very least minimized, by clinicians obtaining comprehensive medical and psychiatric histories of patients before prescribing psychotropics and remaining aware of the genetic and psychosocial factors that may complicate a patient's presentation. Special attention must always be given to remaining aware of the basic effects of aging on the bioavailability and metabolism of medications. In the elderly, in general, medications should be started at lower doses and titrated to higher doses very slowly. Medications that have a particularly complicated side-effect profile in the geriatric population, such as benzodiazepines, tricyclic antidepressants, or neuroleptics, should be used with extreme caution and avoided whenever possible. These considerations can often reduce, or even completely prevent, the risk of adverse effects.

As a greater percentage of the population continues to age and require effective psychotropic medications for the management of common neuropsychiatric conditions, there is an ever-burgeoning need for continued research into the efficacy and safety of pharmacotherapy options in this population.

CLINICS CARE POINTS

---

1. Potentially inappropriate medication use in elderly individuals:
   a. Benzodiazepines and other sedative hypnotics (zolpidem).
   b. Anticholinergic medications (tricyclic antidepressants, paroxetine, diphenhydramine).
   c. Muscle relaxants, nonsteroidal antiinflammatory drugs, and peripheral alpha-1 blockers (prazosin).
2. Understanding pharmacodynamics and pharmacokinetics of medications. Start low and go slow.
3. Obtaining comprehensive medical and psychiatric histories of patients before prescribing psychotropics.
4. Avoid polypharmacy (more than 3 central nervous system active drugs) due to drug-drug and drug-disease interactions.

DISCLOSURE

The authors have nothing to disclose.

REFERENCES

1. The Rural Health Information Hub (HRSA; US HHS). (n.d.). Demographic changes and aging population – rhihub aging in place toolkit. Demographic Changes and Aging Population – RHIhub Aging in Place Toolkit. Retrieved from https://www.ruralhealthinfo.org/toolkits/aging/1/demographics. March 1, 2022.
2. Centers for Disease Control and Prevention. (2021). Depression is not a normal part of growing older. Centers for Disease Control and Prevention. Available at: https://www.cdc.gov/aging/depression/index.html. March 1, 2022.

3. Alzheimer's Association. (2022). 2022 Alzheimer's Disease Facts and Figures. Alzheimers Dement 2022;18. Available at: https://www.alz.org/media/Documents/alzheimers-facts-and-figures.pdf. March 1, 2022

4. Carrarini C, Russo M, Dono F, et al. Agitation and dementia: prevention and treatment strategies in acute and chronic conditions. Front Neurol 2021;12:644317.

5. Tierney J. Practical issues in geriatric psychopharmacology. J Indian Med Assoc 1999;97(4):145–7.

6. Croke L. Beers criteria for inappropriate medication use in older patients: an update from the AGS. Am Fam Physician 2020;101(1):56–7.

7. Naranjo CA, Herrmann N, Mittmann N, et al. Recent advances in geriatric psychopharmacology. Drugs Aging 1995;7(3):184–202.

8. Tillmann J, Reich A. Psychopharmacology and pharmacokinetics. Handb Clin Neurol 2019;167:37–56.

9. Cadieux RJ. Geriatric psychopharmacology. A primary care challenge. Postgrad Med 1993;93(4):281–2, 285-8, 294-282.

10. Catterson ML, Preskorn SH, Martin RL. Pharmacodynamic and pharmacokinetic considerations in geriatric psychopharmacology. Psychiatr Clin North Am 1997;20(1):205–18.

11. Waade RB, Molden E, Refsum H, et al. Serum concentrations of antidepressants in the elderly. Ther Drug Monit 2012;34(1):25–30.

12. Ozdemir V, Fourie J, Busto U, et al. Pharmacokinetic changes in the elderly. Do they contribute to drug abuse and dependence? Clin Pharmacokinet 1996;31(5):372–85.

13. Sommer BR, Fenn H, Pompei P, et al. Safety of antidepressants in the elderly. Expert Opin Drug Saf 2003;2(4):367–83.

14. Farlow MR, Somogyi M. Transdermal patches for the treatment of neurologic conditions in elderly patients: a review. Prim Care Companion CNS Disord 2011;13(6). https://doi.org/10.4088/PCC.11r01149.

15. Meyers BS, Kalayam B. Update in geriatric psychopharmacology. Adv Psychosom Med 1989;19:114–37.

16. Petrie WM, Ban TA. Psychopharmacology for the elderly. Prog Neuropsychopharmacol 1981;5(4):335–42.

17. Wise MG, Tierney J. Psychopharmacology in the elderly. J La State Med Soc 1992;144(10):471–6.

18. Herrmann N. Use of SSRIs in the elderly: obvious benefits but unappreciated risks. Can J Clin Pharmacol 2000;7(2):91–5.

19. Alexopoulos GS, Streim J, Carpenter D, et al. Expert consensus panel for using antipsychotic drugs in older patients. using antipsychotic agents in older patients. J Clin Psychiatry 2004;65(Suppl 2):5–99 [discussion: 100-102, quiz: 103-4].

20. Dorsey ER, Rabbani A, Gallagher SA, et al. Impact of FDA black box advisory on antipsychotic medication use. Arch Intern Med 2010;170(1):96–103.

21. Pratt CE, Davis SM. Divalproex sodium therapy in elderly with dementia-related agitation. Ann Pharmacother 2002;36(10):1625–8.

22. Hsiao SH, Hwang TJ, Lin FJ, et al. The association between the use of cholinesterase inhibitors and cardiovascular events among older patients with Alzheimer disease. Mayo Clin Proc 2021;96(2):350–62.

23. Defilippi JL, Crismon ML. Drug interactions with cholinesterase inhibitors. Drugs Aging 2003;20(6):437–44.

24. Levy HB. Non-benzodiazepine hypnotics and older adults: what are we learning about zolpidem? Expert Rev Clin Pharmacol 2014;7(1):5–8.

Comorbidity and Management of Concurrent Psychiatric and Medical Disorders

Thomas A. Bayer, MD[a,b,*], Ryan Van Patten, PhD[c,d],
Dylan Hershkowitz, MD[d], Gary Epstein-Lubow, MD[d,e,f],
James L. Rudolph, MD SM[a,b,e]

KEYWORDS

- Geriatrics • Multiple chronic conditions • Comanagement • Collaborative care
- Comorbidity • Multimorbidity • Co-occurring conditions • Psychiatry

KEY POINTS

- Psychiatric and medical disorders co-occur commonly in older adults, leading to worse quality of life.
- Evidence-based assessment tools can aid in the identification of suspected delirium, depression, and dementia in older adults with medical disorders who present with psychiatric symptoms including changes in mood or cognition.
- Care coordination, colocation, and collaborative care can improve treatment in older adults with depression or dementia co-occurring with one or more medical disorders.

INTRODUCTION

Aging increases susceptibility to the co-occurrence of medical and psychiatric disorders through multifarious processes ranging from molecular to societal. Biological mechanisms including telomere shortening, epigenetic changes, and cellular senescence underlie susceptibility to multiple diseases spanning multiple organ systems, including the brain.[1,2] In some older adults, social aspects of aging such as loneliness and isolation also accompany increasing disease susceptibility in advanced age, further influencing biological processes via health-damaging behaviors such as poor nutrition and sedentariness.[3] Due in part to these overlapping mechanisms, older

[a] Long-term Services and Supports Center of Innovation, Providence VA Medical Center, 353-373 Niagara St., Providence, RI 02907, USA; [b] Division of Geriatrics and Palliative Medicine, Alpert Medical School of Brown University, 593 Eddy St., POB 438, Providence, RI 02903, USA; [c] Providence VA Medical Center, 830 Chalkstone Ave, Providence, RI 02908, USA; [d] Department of Psychiatry and Human Behavior, Alpert Medical School of Brown University, 593 Eddy Street, APC9 Providence, RI 02903, USA; [e] Department of Health Services, Policy and Practice, Brown University School of Public Health, 121 S. Main Street, Providence, RI 02903, USA; [f] Butler Hospital, 345 Blackstone Blvd, Providence, RI 02906, USA
* Corresponding author.
E-mail address: thomas_bayer@brown.edu

Psychiatr Clin N Am 45 (2022) 745–763
https://doi.org/10.1016/j.psc.2022.07.006
0193-953X/22/Published by Elsevier Inc.

adults with multiple chronic physical health conditions frequently present with psychiatric symptoms that interact in complex ways with co-occurring medical disorders. Critically, optimal treatment of co-occurring physical and mental health conditions requires providers to recognize and address the symptoms concurrently. Isolation, functional decline, caregiver distress, and excess use of acute medical services may result if mental health conditions are overlooked.

Older adults with psychiatric disorders who present to primary care clinics may not receive appropriate or effective care due to under-recognition of mental disorders and the lack of availability of specialty care (eg, psychiatry and psychology). For example, depression co-occurs and interacts with common medical disorders such as Type 2 diabetes, coronary artery disease, heart failure, and chronic obstructive pulmonary disease, often requiring the involvement of multiple specialists. In addition, Alzheimer's disease and related dementias (ADRD) co-occur with depression, anxiety, and chronic medical disorders. Loss of cognitive ability in ADRD ultimately leads to loss of independence for instrumental activities of daily living, which greatly complicates medical decision-making and management of complex medical conditions. Importantly, there is a bidirectional relationship between many physical and emotional/cognitive conditions, where declining physical health can precipitate mental health symptoms (eg, depression and anxiety), and an emotional or cognitive condition can worsen physical health (eg, amotivation due to depression can worsen obesity). This article describes the epidemiology of medical and psychiatric comorbidity in older adults, an approach to assessment, and evidence regarding innovative models of care for dementia and depression in primary care settings.

CASE STUDY
Case Presentation

Ms. A is an 85-year-old widowed woman who presents to her primary care physician's office with red and swollen legs. Her son drives her to the office and she enters the examination room by herself, with visibly labored breathing, and relying on the medical assistant to help her with balance. She reports leg swelling that has been present for two days and states that she does not have shortness of breath. Recently, she has been spending most of her time home alone, for fear of contracting COVID-19. She does not experience hallucinations. She states that her son lives with her and occasionally picks a few items up from the store on her behalf. She reports independence in all of her basic and instrumental activities of daily living but does not recall the last meal she prepared. When asked about sleep, she says that she naps frequently. Her medical history includes hypertension, stage 3 chronic kidney disease, and diet-controlled diabetes. She does not recall with certainty the names or dosing instructions of her medications, and she also forgets the names of friends and relatives sometimes. She has prescriptions for amlodipine and losartan and has intermittently obtained 7-day prescriptions for furosemide throughout the past 2 years for management of edema, most recently 2 months ago. She has never had an echocardiogram. On examination, her blood pressure is 177/92, heart rate 95, and respiratory rate 24. She has bibasilar rales and bilateral 3+ pitting edema of the lower extremities. She asks if she can have a pill to make the leg swelling go away, and she would like to know why she has been so tired.

Discussion

The Creating Age-Friendly Health Systems Initiative names identification, treatment, and management of dementia, depression, and delirium as essential high-level interventions for quality care of older adults. Nine such essential interventions compose four categories: mobility, medications, mentation, and what matters.[4] This "four M" framework of interconnected concepts can help clinicians understand and treat complex problems presenting in older adults who seek medical care.[5] Mrs. A, the patient in the vignette, interconnects elements of each of the "four M's:" She shows obvious mobility difficulty, she has forgotten her medications, and she reports cognitive difficulty and social isolation. Appropriate time and attention to what matters to her would likely uncover important concerns beyond edema and fatigue. Mrs. A's fatigue may result from a medical disorder such as congestive heart failure, a psychiatric disorder such as depression, or both. She may also benefit from a cognitive screening because of concerning memory symptoms.

The tendency to distinguish between medical and psychiatric disorders often reflects historical, cultural, and institutional patterns rather than clean biological distinctions. This is exemplified in a traditional allopathic medical model by the distinction between traditional neurological and traditional psychiatric conditions, both of which occur because of brain dysfunction and both of which involve frequent cognitive, behavioral, and emotional symptoms.[6] In addition, research funding historically followed a "neck up/neck down" isolation and only recently began to recognize the importance of a unified model.[7] An alternative framework is the biopsychosocial model,[8,9] which is interdisciplinary in nature and considers interactions between biological (eg, hormone levels), psychological (eg, mood, affect), and environmental (eg, social support) mechanisms of disease.

The biopsychosocial model has been applied to the understanding and treatment of multiple medical-psychiatric comorbidities, including chronic pain and substance use,[10] diabetes and depression,[11] and cardiovascular symptoms and anxiety,[12] among others. Several mechanistic pathways likely play a role in the mind–body connection, with the most well-known being the hypothalamic–pituitary–adrenal (HPA) axis. Perceived stress, a psychological process, leads to a biological cascade that culminates in the widespread release of glucocorticoids. Chronic exposure to these stress hormones has been associated with a variety of poor health outcomes such as cardiovascular disease,[13] Alzheimer's disease,[14] and periodontal disease.[15] Given the long-term relationship between stress/anxiety and physical conditions, this often manifests as medical-psychiatric comorbidity in later life.[16,17]

EPIDEMIOLOGY

With advancing age, psychiatric disorders increasingly tend to co-occur with medical disorders. In data from a registry of 1,751,841 patients in Scotland, the odds of a mental disorder increased with age, economic deprivation, and number of physical disorders.[18] In this sample, physical–mental comorbidity occurred at a rate of 12.4% in people aged 45 to 64 years, 17.5% in people aged 65 to 84 years, and 30.8% in people 85 years and older. Prevalence of mental–physical comorbidity also increased with economic deprivation, suggesting that older adults of lower socioeconomic status bear a disproportionate comorbidity burden. Clinicians caring for older adults should consider advanced age and low socioeconomic status as important risk factors for medical and psychiatric comorbidity in general.

Knowledge of demographic and socioeconomic trends in the co-occurrence of medical and psychiatric disorders has begun to influence governmental organizations such as the Center for Medicare and Medicaid Services (CMS). In a CMS study of 5.3 million beneficiaries dually enrolled in Medicare and Medicaid in 2008, mental health conditions co-occurred in 39% of those with medical conditions.[19] The same study found that medical cost per month tends to increase with an increasing variety of co-occurring medical conditions.

Descriptive studies of comorbidity or multimorbidity must in some way address the potential for the combinatorial explosion of disease pairs, triads, and clusters. Studies can narrow the focus to a specific combination of diseases or to one disease in combination with many diseases. A useful description of the overall impact of multimorbidity in the population calls for a more complete summary. Aiming for precisely this type of description, a systematic review of disease pairs and cluster prevalence in older adults found 8 studies on depression co-occurring with other disorders.[20] Depression and hypertension occurred together with a prevalence of 1.2% to 12.9%; for depression and heart failure, 0.7% to 0.8%. In one included study, a survey of 1801 US adults over 60 years old with major depression or dysthymia found hypertension in 57.9%, chronic pain in 56.8%, and arthritis in 55.6%.[21] Four studies reported on dementia, reporting a prevalence of dementia combined with hypertension at 2.9% to 5.5%. Record review and clinical evaluation of 3013 patients in a multisite US primary care practice found that among patients with dementia: 82% had hypertension, 39% had diabetes mellitus, and 21% had coronary artery disease. People with and without dementia had similar numbers of comorbidities and rates of specific comorbidities[22] In descriptive studies overviewing multimorbidity as a whole, common disorders such as hypertension, depression, and arthritis tend to co-occur commonly, and surveys of primary care populations tend to find very high rates of comorbidity.

In older adults hospitalized in medical, psychiatric, and surgical settings, medical and psychiatric disorders co-occur commonly. In a quality improvement program in the medicine service of a US teaching hospital, prospective chart reviews of 1590 adults found psychiatric comorbidity in 71.4%, with mood disorder present in 37.2%, anxiety disorder in 21.8%, dementia in 13.6%, and delirium in 10.1%.[23] In Australia, a retrospective chart review of 165 admissions to a geriatric psychiatry unit found medical comorbidity in 91.5%, with diabetes and hypertension among the most common.[24] Similar trends occur in surgical inpatients. Analysis of claims from 1168 patients 70 years and older who underwent fracture surgery in a US level I trauma center found psychiatric comorbidity in 44%, where it was associated with unplanned readmission.[25] In a retrospective chart analysis of 174 orthopedic polytrauma patients over age 60, psychiatric disease, present in 134 (77%) of the sample, was associated with a relative risk (95% confidence interval) of 3.22 (1.03–10) of 30-day mortality.[26] Co-occurrence of medical and psychiatric disease impacts the care of older adults during surgical hospitalization. The association between psychiatric comorbidity and adverse outcomes in surgical patients may highlight an opportunity for further research and enhanced interdisciplinary collaboration.

Delirium deserves special consideration among the psychiatric disorders that can co-occur with medical conditions in older adults. Delirium is an acute disturbance in attention/awareness and at least one other area of cognition. It typically results from an underlying medical disorder, medication, substance intoxication, or withdrawal.[27] The most commonly diagnosed psychiatric disorder in the general hospital, delirium occurs in geriatric medical units with a prevalence of 25%, and in intensive care units (ICUs) with a prevalence ranging from 7% to 80%.[28,29] Especially common in older adults because of predisposing factors of cognitive decline, polypharmacy, and underlying medical conditions, delirium may occur as the first noticeable symptom of a severe illness. It also has a bidirectional relationship with dementia, where dementia is more likely following a delirium, and delirium is more likely in patients with dementia (compared with those without dementia). In a prospective multicenter cohort study of 639 hospitalized patients 65 years and older in the Netherlands, patients with delirium

---

Box 1
Tools for assessment of psychiatric symptoms in older adults with comorbid medical disorders

Delirium
- 4 A's Test[33]
- Recognizing Delirium As part of your Routine[35]
- Confusion Assessment Method[77]
- Confusion Assessment Method for the Intensive Care Unit[78]

Cognition
- Montreal Cognitive Assessment[43]
- Mini Mental Status Examination[39]
- Saint Louis University Mental Status exam[44]
- Clock Drawing Test[45]
- Clock-in-a-Box[48,49]
- Mini-Cog[47]

Depression
- Patient Health Questionnaire 2 and 9[50]
- Geriatric Depression Scale[50]
- Two Question Screen[50]
- Cornell Scale for Depression in Dementia[50]

Anxiety
- General Anxiety Disorder 7[55]
- Hospital Anxiety and Depression Scale[55]

---

were twice as likely to die in the year after hospitalization, and twice as likely to have a poor outcome.[30] Clinicians treating older adults in hospital settings should know when to suspect delirium and how to evaluate it (see below). Clinicians treating older adults in outpatient settings must rule out acute, reversible causes for mental health disorders.[27]

APPROACH
Delirium Assessment

Delirium is primarily a disorder of attention/awareness. Circadian rhythm is often disturbed, with sleep/wake cycle abnormalities that contribute to the difficulty with attention. Symptoms can appear similar to those of many other psychiatric conditions, including anxiety, depression, psychosis, mania, and dementia. The differential diagnosis for underlying causes of delirium includes all of the primary medical disorders and environmental and social changes. Hypoactive delirium is commonly misdiagnosed as depression. Among inpatient psychiatric consultations for depression in older adults, approximately 40% were determined to be delirium, not depression.[31] Dementia is also often confused with delirium, with the difference being the suddenness of the onset (chronic for dementia and acute for delirium) and the severe inattention/lack of awareness that characterizes delirium. Approximately 50% of patients with delirium are found to have comorbid dementia, raising concerns for additional memory aftercare in individuals diagnosed with delirium.[32] Identifying and treating the underlying toxic, metabolic, substance-induced, and/or infectious drivers will assist with the resolution of delirium and can prevent additional adverse health outcomes.

Screening for delirium can be performed quickly. Although psychiatrists and neurologists may be most familiar with identifying delirium through clinical training, multiple screening tools are available to assist providers in identifying delirium with significantly less training. Among these are the 4A's Test for delirium (4AT), Confusion Assessment Method (CAM), the Confusion Assessment Method for the ICU (CAM-ICU) for the critical care setting, and the Recognizing Acute Delirium as part of your Routine (RADAR) scale (**Box 1**). The 4AT scale has a sensitivity of approximately 87% and specificity of 80% when administered among individuals with diverse backgrounds and medical comorbidities.[33] As a test that takes approximately less than 2 min to administer, it is a reasonable and accessible screening tool. The CAM is another tool available for screening for delirium with a sensitivity of 82% and a specificity of 99%.[34] However, this tool requires specific training to complete and takes approximately 10 min at the bedside, which may limit its appeal. In the critical care setting, the CAM-ICU is an abbreviated version that requires less time to administer and has similarly high levels of sensitivity and specificity, at 81% and 98%, respectively.[34] The RADAR is a rapid assessment tool that takes seconds to complete. Although the sensitivity and specificity are lower, at 73% and 67%, respectively, the fact that this tool is easily administered in seconds may broaden its appeal.[35]

Once delirium is identified, a prompt search for the driving pathology and treatment will assist in recovery. It is important to note, however, that deficits persist for quite some time following resolution of the acute syndrome, with cognitive deficits described up to 12 months after discharge from critical illness delirium.[36] Importantly, diagnosis of the psychiatric disease usually requires that potentially reversible causes of cognitive impairment, such as delirium, be addressed first.

Approach to Dementia

In contrast to the acute cognitive change in delirium, the presentation of dementia is more insidious. Delirium is more often observed in the inpatient setting, whereas dementia presents in either inpatient or outpatient domains. Dementia is a descriptive, "umbrella" term that does not imply a particular etiology; symptoms are manifold and can involve numerous aspects of cognitive functioning. Changes in cognitive status observed by the patient or reported in conversation with family members or caregivers warrant cognitive screening and screening for medical and psychiatric drivers. If a treatable cause exists, prompt recognition and treatment can prevent a reversible cause (such as a nutritional deficiency) from progressing to an irreversible state. Similarly, dementia is often misdiagnosed as a primary psychiatric condition. Depression, apathy, and behavioral disturbances are reported in approximately 30% of patients with dementia, leading to the potential for consideration of primary psychiatric pathology instead of a progressive, irreversible neurocognitive disorder.[37] In addition to the potential for a misdiagnosis, anxiety is often part of the clinical picture in dementia and may be a prodromal symptom.[38]

Numerous screening and diagnostic tools exist for the detection and classification of dementia. Of the tools more easily accessible for the general medical or psychiatric setting, the mini-mental state examination (MMSE) and the Montreal Cognitive Assessment (MoCA) are the most widely used.[39] The MMSE has utility in both the inpatient and outpatient settings. It is brief, easily administered, and can assist in monitoring the progression of dementia over time. Drawbacks to the MMSE include its limited ability to diagnose mild cognitive impairment (MCI), poor differentiation of focal deficits, and its limited ability to assess for dysexecutive symptoms. The MoCA, by contrast, is a longer test (approximately 10 min to administer) that shows a better ability to recognize MCI and can provide an abbreviated screening of several cognitive domains.[40–42] It is easily performed at the bedside or in the outpatient setting. However, the MoCA now requires users to undergo training and registration, which may limit its accessibility.[43] The Saint Louis University Mental Status exam is similar to the MoCA and MMSE in length and ease of administration and performs well as a screening tool for MCI and dementia.[44] Providers and researchers can use the test without special training or paying a fee.

The clock drawing test is a screening measure of attention, visuospatial construction, and executive functions.[45] Because clock drawing requires the integration of multiple functional domains, it can be difficult to determine the affected cognitive domain if a patient performs poorly. However, the test can function well as a rapid cognitive screening instrument.[46] The mini-cog exam combines a clock-drawing test with a delayed three-item recall, providing comparable performance to the MMSE with the advantages of brevity and ease of administration.[47] A modified clock drawing test, the "clock-in-the-box" test, typically takes 1–2 min to administer, and has been tested in hospitalized and community-dwelling older adults.[48,49]

If diagnostic uncertainty remains after the cognitive screening, and/or for a more complete understanding of the individual's cognitive status, neuropsychological evaluations may be beneficial. Examples of specific clinical questions relevant to older adults that can be answered by neuropsychologists include (a) determining the extent of cognitive decline, (b) characterizing clinical symptom profiles that align with particular neurodegenerative conditions (eg, behavioral variant frontotemporal dementia versus Alzheimer's disease), (c) identifying primary contributors to cognitive decline (eg, cerebrovascular disease, psychiatric conditions, polypharmacy, sleep apnea), (d) recommending particular cognitive and mental health treatments, and (e) informing decisions about capacity and transitions to higher levels of care. Although trained as psychologists, neuropsychologists typically operate in medical settings and function well in interdisciplinary teams tasked with managing concurrent medical and psychiatric disorders. Therefore, neuropsychological evaluations can be an important component of high-quality care for concurrent physical and mental health conditions.

Mood and Anxiety Symptoms in Patients with Medical Disorders

Mood and anxiety symptoms are also common in the geriatric population, both inpatient and outpatient. The prevalence of depression among older adults is estimated to be between 10% and 20% of the general geriatric population and up to 44% among older adults living in residential care settings.[50] Physical symptoms among depressed and anxious adults may be prominent and are among the most common presenting symptoms of these conditions. By some estimates, more than two-thirds of anxious or depressed adults presenting to primary care may report only physical symptoms.[51]

Overlap between mood/anxiety symptoms and physical concerns presents a challenge for the geriatrician, as one does not want to misattribute a somatic concern to a primary psychiatric disorder and miss an underlying physical illness. Similarly, excessive medical testing and treatments for somatic symptoms presenting secondary to a psychiatric illness may cause harm as well. Somatic symptoms that remain unexplained after an adequate medical workup, however, are more likely to be psychiatric, even if not meeting the full criteria for a diagnostic and statistical manual diagnosis.[51] In addition to this potential diagnostic dilemma, older adults often have medical conditions that can be comorbid with depressive or anxious symptoms. Reduced energy or poor sleep, for example, may be symptoms related to a mood disorder, any number of medical illnesses, or both. Thom and colleagues[52] review the commonly overlapping symptoms between depression and primary medical symptoms. They discuss several frameworks for evaluating depressive symptoms in medical illness. An inclusive approach considers all physical symptoms as potential evidence for major depressive disorder, even if a known medical illness might better account for them. An exclusive approach to diagnosis ignores physical symptoms in the assessment of depression. Finally, a substitutive approach assesses an expanded range of affective symptoms such as pessimism and social withdrawal in place of the excluded physical symptoms. Lacking definitive evidence to support either the inclusive, exclusive, or substitutive approach over the others, clinicians must unexplained symptoms in the context of overall health, environment, and function.

Comprehensive geriatric assessment (CGA), evaluating older adults along multiple domains of health, will help older adults with unexplained or ambiguous symptoms arrive at a pragmatic and person-centered treatment plan. CGA evaluates core domains of functional status, gait speed, cognition, mood, nutritional status, comorbidity, polypharmacy, geriatric syndromes, social support, financial concerns, environmental adequacy, and advance care planning.[53] Implementation of CGA requires a team including a physician, nurse, and social worker, and can include other professions such as pharmacist and occupational therapist. The intervention proceeds stepwise through data-gathering, discussion, treatment plan development, implementation, monitoring, and plan revision.[54] By aiming to understand disease in the context of function and adaptation, the CGA helps to prioritize treatments that align with patient goals and may identify opportunities to improve health status through access to community resources or by discontinuing treatments that do not align with patient goals. In addition to the multidisciplinary approach, CGA relies on evidence-based assessment tools in multiple domains, including mood and anxiety.

Screening Tools for Depression and Anxiety

Many screening tools are available for psychiatric symptoms in the geriatric population. For depression, the Patient Health Questionnaire (PHQ) 2 , PHQ-9, Geriatric Depression Scale (GDS), the Two Question Screen, and the Cornell Scale for Depression in Dementia (CSDD) all have good evidence for sensitivity and specificity.[50] Of these, the Two Question Screen and the PHQ-2 have similar sensitivity, though less specificity, to the other depression screening tools and are much quicker to administer. For anxiety, the GAD-7 and Hospital Anxiety and Depression Scale (HADS) are easy to administer and effective in identifying anxiety symptoms.[55] As anxiety can be a predictor of progressing to develop dementia, screening for anxiety symptoms is important and may suggest lowering the threshold for further cognitive screening.[38]

Case Presentation

Ms. A completed high school and 2 years of college before working as a bank teller until she married and had children. She does not use alcohol or drugs and has never used alcohol to excess. She scores 7 on the GDS, suggesting depression. She is not suicidal. She scores 19 on the Saint Louis University Mental Status Exam, a positive dementia screen. She misses points for day and year, incorrect change, naming only six animals, recalling only 1 out of 5 objects, and incorrect clock drawing test.

Ms. A allows her son to come into the room, who reluctantly shares that he has been doing all of the household shopping for about a year. They mostly eat take-out food from restaurants, and he has hired someone to clean the house. Ms. A has given up driving, and he no longer allows her to do laundry for fear that she may fall down the stairs. He began assisting her with these things after her husband died 2 years ago. He does not administer Ms. A's medications and he insists that she can handle that herself.

CURRENT EVIDENCE

Care model innovations address the complexity of caring for older adults with medical and psychiatric comorbidity by supporting high-quality care. Care coordination, colocation, and collaborative care all aim to improve the treatment of depression or dementia in familiar care settings such as primary care clinics. In care coordination, a nurse or social worker provides proactive communication and behavioral interventions. In colocation, a social worker or psychologist delivers mental health care in the same physical location where patients receive primary care. Care coordination and colocation can each stand-alone or can accompany other components such as enhanced interprofessional communication and team-based care in the case of collaborative care. Collaborative care incorporates care coordination into a structured team-based approach, sometimes featuring colocation or home visits, and aiming to facilitate a true collaboration between the primary care provider and the care manager. These models of care support primary care providers in comprehensively caring for older adults with medical and psychiatric comorbidity. They innovate on conventional patterns of primary care delivery by proactively monitoring patients' status, offering behavioral interventions, and systematically promoting high-quality care. This review will describe care coordination, colocation, and collaborative care in relation to depression and dementia, the two most prevalent disorders occurring concurrently with medical disorders in older adults.

Care Coordination

Care coordination assists older adults with medical and psychiatric comorbidities by proactively communicating with patients and their caregivers and promoting behavioral interventions. Care coordination can function as a stand-alone intervention; in care coordination, a case manager from a nursing, social work, or other professional background helps to organize and facilitate the care of a chronic condition through regular communication with a patient, their health care providers, and potentially their family or other caregivers.

Care coordination improves dementia-related behaviors and caregiver-reported burden in randomized clinical trials. In one systematic review and meta-analysis that included 14 randomized controlled trials (RCTs), coordinating interventions improved patient behavior on the neuropscyhiatric inventory and caregiver burden, and case managers with nursing backgrounds were more effective than case managers from other professional backgrounds at improving caregiver quality of life. Interventions using unsupervised case managers were more effective than those including case manager supervision at reducing the number of patients who are institutionalized.[56]

Care coordination can improve depression symptoms in patients with depression and concurrent medical illness. In a systematic review of 15 RCTs, care coordination interventions that targeted patients with depression and a specific chronic medical illness improved depression symptoms consistently and sometimes improved medical outcomes.[57] In a 2022 systematic review of six studies, telephone-based care management inconsistently improved psychiatric outcomes in populations with a high prevalence of depression.[58] In a pragmatic RCT of transitional care in 127 older adults with multiple chronic conditions and depressive symptoms, nurse care management after hospital discharge did not improve mental function, physical function, depression symptoms, anxiety, or health care costs.[59] Among care management trials for depression, interventions targeting individuals with depression and at least one specific medical illness have showed the most consistent benefit, especially on the outcome of depression symptoms.

Colocation

In the colocation model of integrated care, a mental health care specialist such as a social worker, psychologist, or psychiatric nurse delivers care in the same physical location where patients receive primary medical care.[60] Published evidence supports this model in the treatment of depression, but we did not locate any reports describing this model in dementia care. The Primary Care Research in Substance Abuse and Mental Health for Elders (PRIME-E) randomized 1,390 primary care patients 65 years and older with depression into colocation or enhanced referral. Integrated care increased the odds of the primary outcome of treatment engagement, defined as attendance of an appointment with a mental health provider. It also decreased the time between referral and mental health appointments.[61] Colocation and enhanced referral produced equivalent depression scale outcomes in the overall group of patients with depression. In patients with major depressive disorder, enhanced referral led to greater improvements in the depression scale outcome.[62]

Collaborative Care

In the collaborative model of care, an interprofessional team works in concert with a primary care provider by adding care coordination, anticipatory guidance, and sometimes psychotherapy or medication management (**Fig. 1**). Models of collaborative care vary in the composition of the team, the modality of treatments delivered, and the degree of protocolization of care. Collaborative care interventions in the depression tend to emphasize a treatment algorithm, whereas collaborative care for dementia tends to take a more flexible approach to support caregivers through education on nonpharmacologic approaches to dementia-related behaviors such as resistance to care. Collaborative care models always engage a multidisciplinary team in the management of a specific type of clinical problem, and they tend to function as a support structure for primary care providers. They tend to emphasize regular follow-up and they usually contain a structured approach to assessment and/or treatment.[61] Primary care providers working in collaborative care models remain engaged in managing depression or dementia collaboratively alongside other clinical problems which they may manage independently or through a more traditional referral-based model of care.

A systematic review of 29 studies of collaborative care for older adults with psychiatric disorders found that collaborative care can improve clinical outcomes in

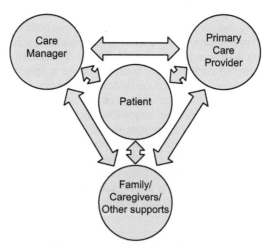

Fig. 1. Collaborative care of dementia or depression features a care manager, typically a nurse, social worker, or nurse practitioner. The family caregiver plays a key role in dementia care, less so in the collaborative care of depression. The care manager provides disease-specific counseling and behavioral interventions and collaborates with the primary care provider and patient–caregiver dyad in the development of a treatment plan.

depression in a variety of clinical settings and can be cost-effective. Only two of the studies evaluated collaborative care for dementia in less than 600 total participants. Collaborative care increased the use of cholinesterase inhibitors in both studies. In one, it also reduced neuropsychiatric symptoms, and in the other, it improved adherence to treatment guidelines.[63]

Multiple clinical trials support the use of collaborative care in the treatment of depression in older adults. A multisite trial randomized 1801 patients with major depressive disorder aged 60 years and older to usual care or the Improving Mood-Promoting Access to Collaborative Treatment (IMPACT) intervention. Participants had an average of three chronic diseases, and 65% had chronic pain. In IMPACT, a nurse or psychologist functioned as a care manager and delivered an intake visit at the primary care site where they educated the patient and elicited treatment preferences. The care managers met regularly with a psychiatrist and a liaison primary care physician to discuss the cases. Incorporating patient preferences and a treatment algorithm, the care managers recommended a treatment plan to the patient's primary care provider who would incorporate the recommendations at their discretion. The algorithm emphasized the use of selective serotonin reuptake inhibitors (SSRIs) as first-line pharmacotherapy, and Problem Solving Treatment in Primary Care, a structured psychotherapeutic intervention that the care managers could deliver at the primary care site. Compared with participants in usual care, participants receiving the IMPACT intervention were more likely to receive, respond to, and be satisfied with depression treatment, and experienced greater reductions in depression severity, greater quality of life, and less functional impairment.[64]

The Prevention Of Suicide in Primary Care Elderly: Clinical Trial (PROSPECT) study randomized 598 patients with depression aged 60 years and older to a collaborative care intervention or usual care. This intervention featured a group of 15 depression care managers consisting of social workers, nurses, and psychologists. The care managers collaborated with the primary care providers by helping them identify depression, recommending algorithm-based pharmacotherapy (SSRI first), monitoring the status of participants, and providing interpersonal psychotherapy to participants who preferred this treatment modality. Care managers met weekly with study psychiatrists. Participants in the intervention group experienced greater reductions in suicidal ideation and higher rates of response to depression treatment at 12 months of follow-up.[65] These benefits continued to accrue after 24 months of follow-up.[66]

The collaborative care model has also improved depression outcomes in clinical trials specific to depression and coronary heart disease. A systematic review and meta-analysis found six randomized trials comparing collaborative care to a control group in participants with depression and coronary heart disease. In the meta-analysis, which included a total of 655 participants, patients in collaborative care achieved remission of depression at higher rates and experienced greater reductions in depression symptoms. Collaborative care did not lead to reductions in major adverse cardiovascular events or all-cause mortality.[67]

The collaborative model of care has undergone a variety of variations and innovations aiming to meet the needs of older adults with ADRD and their caregivers. A narrative review of seven collaborative care models of dementia identifies key characteristics of collaborative dementia care models in the primary care setting.[68] Although collaborative models of depression tend to emphasize orientation toward the treatment preferences of the individual patient, collaborative models of dementia tend to orient toward the needs of the patient–caregiver dyad. Consistent with the dyadic focus, potential treatments offered through collaborative dementia care range from referral to community resources to discontinuation of potentially harmful medications to education about nonpharmacologic strategies for managing difficult dementia-associated behaviors.

Collaborative models of dementia care include a care management role, and the professional background of the care manager varies between models. In the Alzheimer's and Dementia Care (ADC) program, a nurse practitioner fulfills care management functions and also functions as a medical advisor and consultant to the patient–caregiver dyad and the referring provider.[69] In the Aging Brain Care Medical Home, a registered nurse fulfills a care management role on a team that includes social workers.[70] In Alzheimer's Disease Coordinated Care for San Diego Seniors (ACCESS), a social worker provides care management.[71] Outcomes in trials of collaborative dementia care, which vary among studies, include increased adherence to treatment guidelines, decrease in caregiver burden, and decreased utilization of primary care and emergency services.[72] Collaborative dementia care provides a clinical setting adjacent to primary care where a multidisciplinary team can apply specialized expertise to the behavioral problems of dementia. The dementia care team, by addressing dementia-related behavioral concerns, allows the primary care provider to focus more of their visit time on managing chronic medical conditions. Likewise, as the dementia care team works in collaboration with the primary care provider, they are well-positioned to recognize and coordinate intervention when a chronic medical condition requires prompt attention.

Collaborative models of dementia care and related approaches continue to spread through new care environments, adapting to the interests of payers and other stakeholders. In the Care of Persons with Dementia in their Environments (COPE) program, an occupational therapist and advanced practice nurse provide home visits to patient–caregiver dyads. A pragmatic trial compared COPE to usual care in a state and Medicaid-funded home care program. COPE visits provide a personalized treatment plan within a protocol emphasizing specific points such as fall prevention, physical activity, and medication review. Caregivers reported greater wellbeing in the group receiving COPE, and the persons with dementia engaged more in meaningful activities.[72] The COPE program benefits older adults with medical conditions that co-occur with dementia by adding enhanced collaborative dementia care to a specialized home-based primary care program.

Program of All-Inclusive Care for the Elderly

The Program of All-Inclusive Care for the Elderly (PACE) delivers collaborative care bundled with comprehensive and social services to older adults to help them remain in their homes rather than enter nursing homes. Rather than specialize in a specific psychiatric or medical disorder, PACE serves patients who would otherwise qualify for nursing home care. PACE provides primary care, social work, psychiatric and other specialty care, dentistry, meals, prescription drugs, and more, through PACE centers. The program provides transportation to and from the centers, and accommodates the needs of participants who cannot travel to the center or who require a variety of other services.[73] CMS, which provides an administrative framework for individual states to implement PACE, reports programs in 31 states as of June 2021.[74] A systematic review of six studies comparing PACE to other models of care found mixed results regarding functional and mortality outcomes of program participants and found that PACE participants tended to have lower rates of hospitalization and lower length of stay than comparison groups. One included study of the cost found higher costs in PACE compared with the comparison Medicaid waiver program but lower than nursing home costs.[75] When implemented successfully, PACE offers a collaborative care model flexible enough to meet the needs of older adults with almost any combination of medical and psychiatric disorders, provided that the person can be safely cared for at home.

Case Presentation

Ms. A provides a blood sample at the end of the visit, and an EKG shows a normal si-nus rhythm with left ventricular hypertrophy. She leaves with a new prescription for furosemide, an order for an echocardiogram, and instructions to follow-up in 2 weeks. Laboratory tests show stable chronic kidney disease, normal thyroid function, and an elevated NT-Pro-BNP.

She returns in 2 weeks with her son and has not yet scheduled an echocardiogram. Her son hesitates in the corridor outside the exam room and asks if a nurse could visit the home twice per day to administer medications. A nurse care manager instructs Ms. A's son is using a pill box to organize the medications.

At the follow-up visit, she states she has been sleeping better. She no longer ap-pears short of breath. Her blood pressure is 154/7 with a heart rate of 80. Her breath sounds are clear and her lower extremity edema has noticeably decreased. She con-tinues to appear unbalanced when ambulating the corridor of the office. She does not have motor rigidity, and she is able to tap her toes and rapidly move her hands without visible slowness. She undergoes MRI of the brain, which shows diffuse white matter hyperintensities and enlargement of the ventricles.

At a later follow-up visit, she and her son learn that she has dementia, most likely resulting from Alzheimer's disease. Ms. A's son says that she is refusing to take her meds and refusing to bathe. He fears that she will develop heart failure symptoms again if she does not begin taking the medications again. He asks if there is a medi-cation that he could mix into her food that will make her bathe and take her pills. Ms. A and her son accept a referral to a collaborative dementia care program after learning that they will be able to meet regularly with the office's nurse care manager. The care manager will teach Ms. A's son behavioral strategies to encourage her to accept care such as medication and reminders to bathe. They learn that the nurse care manager will be available by telephone between visits to help. They also accept a referral to a home health care agency for a home safety evaluation.

DISCUSSION

Psychiatric disorders, especially depression, delirium, and dementia, frequently occur in combination with medical disorders in older adults. When evaluating an acute change in mental status, medical providers must consider delirium, which occurs in the setting of acute illness and other physiological insults. Providers can use several numerous tools to evaluate for delirium and should undertake a more detailed assess-ment in the case of a positive screen. Depression occurs commonly in the setting of chronic medical illnesses, especially illnesses causing pain and loss of endurance. Depression symptoms can overlap substantially with those of medical illnesses. Thoughtful consideration and careful assessment of symptoms and use of depression screening tools can help to diagnose depression in individuals with high burdens of chronic somatic symptoms. Dementia risk increases greatly with advancing age and medical comorbidities, and symptoms of dementia complicate the management of medical conditions such as heart failure which require self-management.

Care model innovations such as colocation, care coordination, and collaborative care can improve the management of older adults with concurrent psychiatric and medical disorders, especially dementia or depression. Collaborative models of care incorporate care management, enhanced interprofessional communication, and team-based care to deliver multicomponent interventions. These innovations work by enhancing care quality in settings such as primary care clinics in which patients already feel comfortable by promoting behavioral interventions and by enhancing provider availability in dementia care. In depression care, they support screening and diagnosis by primary care providers and then they enhance the availability of psychotherapy while promoting an evidence-based approach to medication management. Efforts are underway to make these models more available, by enhancing mechanisms to pay for all aspects of comprehensive dementia care.[76]

SUMMARY

Depression, delirium, and dementia tend to occur in older adults with medical comorbidities, adding further complications where conventional patterns of care delivery already face overwhelm. Providers across settings can begin to meet this challenge and provide excellent, compassionate, comprehensive care by identifying patients at risk and using evidence-based screening tools to support clinical assessment. Provider groups and health systems can implement care model innovations such as collaborative care to improve the management of older adults with medical disorders and comorbid depression or dementia.

CLINICS CARE POINTS

- Aging confers susceptibility to multimorbidity of disease across organ systems including concurrent medical and psychiatric disorders.
- Evidence-based screening tools aid the assessment of delirium, depression, and dementia, the most common causes of psychiatric symptoms in older adults with medical disorders.
- Care model innovations such as collaborative care, if successfully implemented, enhance the quality of care for dementia and depression in older adults with medical disorders.

DISCLOSURE

The authors have no relevant financial relationships to disclose.
Thomas A Bayer received support from the Veterans Affairs Office of Academic Affiliations during the preparation of this review.

REFERENCES

1. Bishop NA, Lu T, Yankner BA. Neural mechanisms of ageing and cognitive decline. Nature 2010;464(7288):529–35.
2. Barnes PJ. Mechanisms of development of multimorbidity in the elderly. Eur Respir J 2015;45(3):790–806.
3. Fried LP, Carlson MC, Freedman M, et al. A social model for health promotion for an aging population: initial evidence on the Experience Corps model. J Urban Health 2004;81(1):64–78.
4. Mate KS, Berman A, Laderman M, et al. Creating age-friendly health systems - a vision for better care of older adults. Healthc (Amst) 2018;6(1):4–6.
5. Lesser S, Zakharkin S, Louie C, et al. Clinician knowledge and behaviors related to the 4Ms framework of Age-Friendly Health Systems. J Am Geriatr Soc 2022; 70(3):789–800.
6. Searight HR. Psychosocial knowledge and allopathic medicine: points of convergence and departure. J Med Humanit 1994;15(4):221–32.

7. Hernandez AR, Hoffman JM, Hernandez CM, et al. Reuniting the body "neck up and neck down" to understand cognitive aging: the nexus of geroscience and neuroscience. J Gerontol A Biol Sci Med Sci 2022;77(1):e1–9.

8. Engel GL. The need for a new medical model: a challenge for biomedicine. Science 1977;196(4286):129–36.

9. Fava GA, Sonino N. The biopsychosocial model thirty years later. Psychother Psychosom 2007;77(1):1–2. https://doi.org/10.1159/000110052.

10. Cheatle MD, Gallagher RM. Chronic pain and comorbid mood and substance use disorders: a biopsychosocial treatment approach. Curr Psychiatry Rep 2006;8(5):371–6.

11. Habtewold TD, Islam M, Radie YT, et al. Comorbidity of depression and diabetes: an application of biopsychosocial model. Int J Ment Health Syst 2016;10(1):1–9.

12. Sotile WM. Biopsychosocial care of heart patients: are we practicing what we preach? Families, Syst Health 2005;23(4):400–3.

13. Sher L. Type D personality: the heart, stress, and cortisol. Qjm 2005;98(5):323–9.

14. Ennis GE, An Y, Resnick SM, et al. Long-term cortisol measures predict Alzheimer disease risk. Neurology 2017;88(4):371–8.

15. Rosania AE, Low KG, McCormick CM, et al. Stress, depression, cortisol, and periodontal disease. J Periodontol 2009;80(2):260–6.

16. Cohen S, Janicki-Deverts D, Doyle WJ, et al. Chronic stress, glucocorticoid receptor resistance, inflammation, and disease risk. Proc Natl Acad Sci U S A 2012;109(16):5995–9.

17. Gouin JP, Hantsoo L, Kiecolt-Glaser JK. Immune dysregulation and chronic stress among older adults: a review. Neuroimmunomodulation 2008;15(4–6):251–9.

18. Barnett K, Mercer SW, Norbury M, et al. Epidemiology of multimorbidity and implications for health care, research, and medical education: a cross-sectional study. Lancet 2012;380(9836):37–43.

19. Physical and mental health condition prevalence and ... - CMS. CMS.gov.Available at: https://www.cms.gov/Medicare-Medicaid-Coordination/Medicare-and-Medicaid-Coordination/Medicare-Medicaid-Coordination-Office/Downloads/Dual_Condition_Prevalence_Comorbidity_2014.pdf. Published September 2014. Accessed April 15, 2022.

20. Sinnige J, Braspenning J, Schellevis F, et al. The prevalence of disease clusters in older adults with multiple chronic diseases – a systematic literature review. PLoS One 2013;8(11):e79641.

21. Noël PH, Williams JW Jr, Unützer J, et al. Depression and comorbid illness in elderly primary care patients: impact on multiple domains of health status and well-being. Ann Fam Med 2004;2(6):555–62. https://doi.org/10.1370/afm.143.

22. Schubert CC, Boustani M, Callahan CM, et al. Comorbidity profile of dementia patients in primary care: are they sicker? J Am Geriatr Soc 2006;54(1):104–9.

23. Oldham MA, Walsh P, Maeng DD, et al. Integration of a proactive, multidisciplinary mental health team on hospital medicine improves provider and nursing satisfaction. J Psychosom Res 2020;134:110112.

24. Goh AM, Westphal A, Daws T, et al. A retrospective study of medical comorbidities in psychogeriatric patients. Psychogeriatrics 2016;16(1):12–9.

25. Gitajn IL, Titus A, Mastrangelo S, et al. Psychiatric illness is common in elderly fracture patients. J Orthop Trauma 2019;33(3):149–54.

26. Mun F, Ringenbach K, Baer B, et al. Factors influencing geriatric orthopaedic trauma mortality. Injury 2022;53(3):919–24.

27. American Psychiatric Association. Diagnostic and statistical manual of mental disorders. 5th edition. Washington, DC: APA Press; 2013.

28. Inouye SK, Westendorp RG, Saczynski JS. Delirium in elderly people. Lancet 2014;383(9920):911–22.

29. National institute for health and care excellence: delirium: prevention, diagnosis and management. NICE Clinical guidelines 103. london, national institute for health and care excellence. 2010. Available at. https://www.nice.org.uk/guidance/cg103/evidence/full-guideline-pdf-134653069. Accessed March 27, 2022.

30. Buurman BM, Hoogerduijn JG, de Haan RJ, et al. Geriatric conditions in acutely hospitalized older patients: prevalence and one-year survival and functional decline. PLoS One 2011;6(11):e26951.

31. Farrell KR, Ganzini L. Misdiagnosing delirium as depression in medically ill elderly patients. Arch Intern Med 1995;155(22):2459–64.

32. Bellelli G, Morandi A, Di Santo SG, et al. "Delirium Day": a nationwide point prevalence study of delirium in older hospitalized patients using an easy standardized diagnostic tool. BMC Med 2016;14:106.

33. De J, Wand APF, Smerdely PI, et al. Validating the 4A's test in screening for delirium in a culturally diverse geriatric inpatient population. Int J Geriatr Psychiatry 2017;32(12):1322–9.

34. Shi Q, Warren L, Saposnik G, et al. Confusion assessment method: a systematic review and meta-analysis of diagnostic accuracy. Neuropsychiatr Dis Treat 2013; 9:1359–70.

35. Voyer P, Champoux N, Desrosiers J, et al. Recognizing acute delirium as part of your routine [RADAR]: a validation study. BMC Nurs 2015;14:19.

36. Pandharipande PP, Girard TD, Jackson JC, et al. Long-term cognitive impairment after critical illness. N Engl J Med 2013;369(14):1306–16.

37. Lyketsos CG, Lopez O, Jones B, et al. Prevalence of neuropsychiatric symptoms in dementia and mild cognitive impairment: results from the cardiovascular health study. JAMA 2002;288(12):1475–83.

38. Gimson A, Schlosser M, Huntley JD, et al. Support for midlife anxiety diagnosis as an independent risk factor for dementia: a systematic review. BMJ Open 2018; 8(4):e019399.

39. Finney GR, Minagar A, Heilman KM. Assessment of mental status. Neurol Clin 2016;34(1):1–16.

40. Ciesielska N, Sokołowski R, Mazur E, et al. Is the Montreal Cognitive Assessment (MoCA) test better suited than the Mini-Mental State Examination (MMSE) in mild cognitive impairment (MCI) detection among people aged over 60? Meta-analysis. Czy test Montreal Cognitive Assessment (MoCA) może być skuteczniejszy od powszechnie stosowanego Mini-Mental State Examination (MMSE) w wykrywaniu łagodnych zaburzeń funkcji poznawczych u osób po 60. roku życia? Metaanaliza. Psychiatr Pol 2016;50(5):1039–52.

41. Hoops S, Nazem S, Siderowf AD, et al. Validity of the MoCA and MMSE in the detection of MCI and dementia in Parkinson disease. Neurology 2009;73(21): 1738–45.

42. Pinto TCC, Machado L, Bulgacov TM, et al. Is the Montreal Cognitive Assessment (MoCA) screening superior to the Mini-Mental State Examination (MMSE) in the detection of mild cognitive impairment (MCI) and Alzheimer's Disease (AD) in the elderly? Int Psychogeriatr 2019;31(4):491–504.

43. Hodges JR. Standardized mental test schedules: their uses and abuses. In: Cognitive assessment for clinicians. 3rd edition. Oxford University Press; 2018. p. 155–7. Chapter.

44. Shwartz SK, Morris RD, Penna S. Psychometric properties of the Saint Louis University Mental Status Examination. Appl Neuropsychol Adult 2019;26(2):101–10.
45. Grande LJ, Rudolph JL, Davis R, et al. Clock drawing: standing the test of time. In: Ashendorf L, Swenson R, Libon D, editors. The boston process approach to neuropsychological assessment: a practitioner's guide. New York: Oxford University Press; 2013. p. 229–48.
46. van der Burg M, Bouwen A, Stessens J, et al. Scoring clock tests for dementia screening: a comparison of two scoring methods. Int J Geriatr Psychiatry 2004; 19(7):685–9.
47. Borson S, Scanlan JM, Chen P, et al. The Mini-Cog as a screen for dementia: validation in a population-based sample. J Am Geriatr Soc 2003;51(10):1451–4.
48. Chester JG, Grande LJ, Milberg WP, et al. Cognitive screening in community-dwelling elders: performance on the clock-in-the-box. Am J Med 2011;124(7): 662–9.
49. Jackson CE, Grande LJ, Doherty K, et al. The Clock-in-the-Box, a brief cognitive screen, is associated with failure to return home in an elderly hospitalized sample. Clin interventions Aging 2016;11:1715–21. https://doi.org/10.2147/CIA.S118235.
50. Tsoi KK, Chan JY, Hirai HW, et al. Comparison of diagnostic performance of Two-Question Screen and 15 depression screening instruments for older adults: systematic review and meta-analysis [published correction appears in Br J Psychiatry. Br J Psychiatry 2017;210(4):255–60.
51. Kapfhammer HP. Somatic symptoms in depression. Dialogues Clin Neurosci 2006;8(2):227–39. https://doi.org/10.31887/DCNS.2006.8.2/hpkapfhammer.
52. Thom R, Silbersweig DA, Boland RJ. Major depressive disorder in medical illness: a review of assessment, prevalence, and treatment options. Psychosom Med 2019;81(3):246–55.
53. Pilotto A, Cella A, Pilotto A, et al. Three decades of comprehensive geriatric assessment: evidence coming from different healthcare settings and specific clinical conditions. J Am Med Dir Assoc 2017;18(2):192. e1-11.
54. Reuben DB, Rosen S, Schickedanz HB. Principles of Geriatric Assessment. In: Halter JB, Ouslander JG, Studenski S, et al, editors. Hazzard's geriatric medicine and gerontology, 7e. McGraw Hill; 2017. Available at: https://accessmedicine. mhmedical.com/content.aspx?bookid=1923&sectionid=144517796. Accessed April 15, 2022.
55. Wetherell JL, Birchler GD, Ramsdell J, et al. Screening for generalized anxiety disorder in geriatric primary care patients. Int J Geriatr Psychiatry 2007;22(2): 115–23.
56. Backhouse A, Ukoumunne OC, Richards DA, et al. The effectiveness of community-based coordinating interventions in dementia care: a meta-analysis and subgroup analysis of intervention components. BMC Health Serv Res 2017;17(1):717.
57. Baker JM, Grant RW, Gopalan A. A systematic review of care management interventions targeting multimorbidity and high care utilization. BMC Health Serv Res 2018;18(1):65.
58. Lim CT, Rosenfeld LC, Nissen NJ, et al. Remote care management for older adult populations with elevated prevalence of depression or anxiety and comorbid chronic medical illness: a systematic review. J Acad Consult Liaison Psychiatry 2022. https://doi.org/10.1016/j.jaclp.2022.02.005.
59. Markle-Reid M, McAiney C, Fisher K, et al. Effectiveness of a nurse-led hospital-to-home transitional care intervention for older adults with multimorbidity and

depressive symptoms: a pragmatic randomized controlled trial. PLoS One 2021; 16(7):e0254573.

60. Bruce ML, Sirey JA. Integrated care for depression in older primary care patients. Can J Psychiatry 2018;63(7):439–46.

61. Bartels SJ, Coakley EH, Zubritsky C, et al. Improving access to geriatric mental health services: a randomized trial comparing treatment engagement with integrated versus enhanced referral care for depression, anxiety, and at-risk alcohol use. Am J Psychiatry 2004;161(8):1455–62.

62. Krahn DD, Bartels SJ, Coakley E, et al. PRISM-E: comparison of integrated care and enhanced specialty referral models in depression outcomes. Psychiatr Serv 2006;57(7):946–53.

63. Dham P, Colman S, Saperson K, et al. Collaborative care for psychiatric disorders in older adults: a systematic review. Can J Psychiatry 2017;62(11):761–71.

64. Unützer J, Katon W, Callahan CM, et al. Collaborative care management of late-life depression in the primary care setting: a randomized controlled trial. JAMA 2002;288(22):2836–45.

65. Bruce ML, Ten Have TR, Reynolds CF 3rd, et al. Reducing suicidal ideation and depressive symptoms in depressed older primary care patients: a randomized controlled trial. JAMA 2004;291(9):1081–91.

66. Alexopoulos GS, Reynolds CF 3rd, Bruce ML, et al. Reducing suicidal ideation and depression in older primary care patients: 24-month outcomes of the PROSPECT study. Am J Psychiatry 2009;166(8):882–90.

67. Tully PJ, Baumeister H. Collaborative care for comorbid depression and coronary heart disease: a systematic review and meta-analysis of randomised controlled trials. BMJ Open 2015;5(12):e009128.

68. Heintz H, Monette P, Epstein-Lubow G, et al. Emerging collaborative care models for dementia care in the primary care setting: a narrative review. Am J Geriatr Psychiatry 2020;28(3):320–30.

69. Reuben DB, Evertson LC, Wenger NS, et al. The university of california at los angeles Alzheimer's and dementia care program for comprehensive, coordinated, patient-centered care: preliminary data. J Am Geriatr Soc 2013;61(12):2214–8.

70. LaMantia MA, Alder CA, Callahan CM, et al. The aging brain care medical home: preliminary data. J Am Geriatr Soc 2015;63(6):1209–13.

71. Vickrey BG, Mittman BS, Connor KI, et al. The effect of a disease management intervention on quality and outcomes of dementia care: a randomized, controlled trial. Ann Intern Med 2006;145(10):713–26.

72. Pizzi LT, Jutkowitz E, Prioli KM, et al. Cost-Benefit Analysis of the COPE Program for Persons Living With Dementia: Toward a Payment Model. Innov Aging 2021; 6(1):igab042.

73. Programs of all-inclusive care for the elderly (PACE). 2011. Available at: https://www.cms.gov/Regulations-and-Guidance/Guidance/Manuals/Downloads/pace111c06.pdf. Accessed April 15, 2022.

74. State website List - Medicaid. Medicaid.gov. 2021. https://www.medicaid.gov/medicaid/ltss/downloads/integrating-care/state-website-list.pdf. Accessed April 15, 2022.

75. Arku D, Felix M, Warholak T, et al. Program of all-inclusive care for the elderly (PACE) versus other programs: a scoping review of health outcomes. Geriatrics (Basel) 2022;7(2):31.

76. Lees Haggerty K, Epstein-Lubow G, Spragens LH, et al. Recommendations to improve payment policies for comprehensive dementia care. J Am Geriatr Soc 2020;68(11):2478–85.

77. Wei LA, Fearing MA, Sternberg EJ, et al. The confusion assessment method: a systematic review of current usage. J Am Geriatr Soc 2008;56(5):823–30.
78. Gusmao-Flores D, Salluh JI, Chalhub RÁ, et al. The confusion assessment method for the intensive care unit (CAM-ICU) and intensive care delirium screening checklist (ICDSC) for the diagnosis of delirium: a systematic review and meta-analysis of clinical studies. Crit Care 2012;16(4):R115.

Geriatric Psychiatry Across the Spectrum

Medical Student, Resident, and Fellow Education

Michelle L. Conroy, MD[a,b,]*, Kirsten M. Wilkins, MD[a,b,1],
Laura I. van Dyck, MD[c,2], Brandon C. Yarns, MD, MS[d,e]

KEYWORDS

- Geriatric psychiatry • Geriatrics • Education • Training • Recruitment

KEY POINTS

- The older adult population is rapidly growing and increasingly diverse.
- The number of physicians pursuing geriatric psychiatry fellowship training is waning.
- Geriatric psychiatry education spans all years of medical training and should be targeted to increase the knowledge base of learners, as well as encourage recruitment into geriatric psychiatry subspecialty training.
- Geriatric psychiatry fellowship training consists of interdisciplinary collaboration and exposure across a range of clinical settings to promote an in depth, detailed understanding of the complexities and nuances in providing care to older adult patients.
- General psychiatrists can access several learning opportunities germane to the treatment of older adult populations.

INTRODUCTION

The US health-care system faces a burgeoning aging population. The US population aged older than 65 years is projected to increase from 40.3 million in 2010 to 83.7 million in 2050.[1,2] A significant number of older adults suffer from mental health or substance use disorders, estimated between 14% and 20%.[3] Mental health needs in

[a] Yale University School of Medicine, 333 Cedar Street, New Haven, CT 06510 USA; [b] VA Connecticut Healthcare System, 950 Campbell Avenue, Psychiatry 116A, West Haven, CT 06516, USA; [c] Mount Sinai School of Medicine, 1 Gustave L. Levy Place, New York, NY 10029, USA; [d] VA Greater Los Angeles Healthcare System, 11301 Wilshire Boulevard, Building 401, 116AE, Los Angeles, CA 90073, USA; [e] University of California, Los Angeles (UCLA), 10833 Le Conte Avenue, Los Angeles, CA 90095, USA
[1] Present address: 2 Parkland Place, Milford, CT 06460.
[2] Present address: 440 East 88th Street, New York, NY 10128.
* Corresponding author. 130 Myren Street, Fairfield, CT 06824.
E-mail address: Michelle.L.Conroy@yale.edu

Psychiatr Clin N Am 45 (2022) 765–777
https://doi.org/10.1016/j.psc.2022.07.008
0193-953X/22/Published by Elsevier Inc.

psych.theclinics.com

aged patients—commonly with comorbid medical and cognitive disorders—present unique challenges in psychiatric diagnosis and treatment.

In addition, the older adult population is projected to significantly increase its racial and ethnic diversity during the next several decades. It is estimated to increase from 20% racial/ethnicity minority in 2010 to 42% minority in 2050.[1] The American Psychological Association indicates the importance for multicultural competency training in caring for the increasingly diverse older population.[4]

Despite the growing need, fewer trainees are entering geriatric subspecialties. Although the number of medical graduates entering psychiatric residencies is increasing, fewer psychiatric resident graduates are pursuing geriatric subspecialties (**Fig. 1**). According to data from the National Resident Matching Program, the number of allopathic medical school seniors and graduates entering psychiatry residency programs has increased from 600 in 2002 to 1188 in 2020, a corresponding increase from 4.3% to 6.3%.[5] However, the number of residents entering geriatric psychiatry fellowships has dwindled compared with that of other psychiatric fellowships, from 106 enrollees in geriatric psychiatry during 2002 to 2003 academic year to 48 during 2020 to 2021.[6] This 55% decline in fellowship enrollment occurred despite a relatively constant number of approximately 60 geriatric psychiatry fellowship programs.[6,7]

The US medical education system has a responsibility to foster recruitment into geriatric subspecialties and to ensure competence in geriatrics across medical specialties in order to meet the complex health demands of an aging population. In this article, we discuss current geriatric psychiatry training requirements, potential strategies of recruitment into the field and educational requirements and opportunities at the medical school, residency, fellowship levels related to the care of older adults.

Medical Student Education

Demographic trends necessitate that virtually all future physicians are trained to care for older adults, many of whom will have mental health concerns. Despite this imperative, there exists no national requirement or standardization for geriatric psychiatry education across undergraduate medical education. The Liaison Committee on Medical Education (LCME), recognized by the US Department of Education to accredit medical schools in the United States and Canada, notes in standard 7.2 that medical curriculum must include "content and clinical experiences related to…each phase of the human life cycle; continuity of care…and end-of-life care."[8] However, there are no

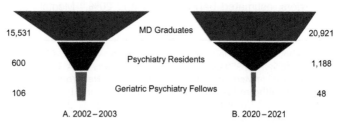

A. 2002–2003   B. 2020–2021

Fig. 1. A Shrinking Number of Trainees Pursuing Geriatric Psychiatry Fellowship: 2002 versus 2020. (*A*) In 2002, 15,531 allopathic medical students graduated in the US (AAMC), 600 US MD seniors and US MD graduates enrolled into psychiatry residency (NRMP), and 106 psychiatry residents enrolled into geriatric psychiatry fellowships. (*B*) In 2020, 20,921 allopathic medical students graduated in the US (AAMC), 1,188 US MD seniors and US MD graduates enrolled into psychiatry residency (NRMP) but only 58 psychiatry residents enrolled into geriatric psychiatry fellowships.

specifications regarding what medical students should be taught in geriatric psychiatry or where and how in the medical curriculum such teaching should take place.

Recognizing the need for all medical students to be trained to provide safe and effective care for older adults, experts in the field made recommendations for medical student education in geriatrics. In 2009, Leipzig and colleagues published the seminal "Do Not Kill Granny" article, which defined the minimum geriatrics competencies all graduating medical students should attain in preparation for internship.[9] Curricular domains include medication management; cognitive and behavioral disorders; self-care capacity; falls, balance, and gait disorders; atypical presentation of disease; palliative care; hospital care for elders; and health-care planning and promotion. These competencies were updated in 2021.[10,11] In 2012, the Institute of Medicine published a report entitled "The Mental Health and Substance Use Workforce for Older Adults: In Whose Hands?," which highlighted the prevalence of mental health concerns among older adults and urged the development of core competencies in geriatric mental health and substance use "for the entire spectrum of personnel who care for older adults."[3] In response to this report and in recognition of a need for more specific medical student competencies in geriatric *mental health*, Lehmann and colleagues published learning objectives for graduating medical students in this area.[12] Domains include normal aging, the assessment of the geriatric patient, principles of psychopharmacology, depression, dementia, and delirium. The authors followed up with recommendations for learner-centered, evidence-informed teaching strategies for each domain and recommendations for where in the 4-year medical school curriculum they might be taught.[13]

Although the above recommendations were circulated and endorsed by national organizations, including the Association of American Medical Colleges (AAMC) and the American Association for Geriatric Psychiatry (AAGP), widespread implementation is contingent on adequate resources, curricular time, and geriatrics expertise, which are often lacking. A national survey of clerkship directors in psychiatry found that 21% of clerkships lacked any specific instruction in geriatric psychiatry.[14] Moreover, with less than 1400 board-certified geriatric psychiatrists in the United States,[15] it is likely that many of the ~20,000 graduating medical students in this country will neither meet nor train under one during their time in medical school. Geriatric psychiatry educators across the country face both challenges and opportunities as medical schools undergo curricular revisions nationwide, integrating courses and clerkships and shrinking dedicated curricular time.[16]

Even in the absence of formal required geriatrics and geriatric psychiatry courses and rotations, faculties passionate about geriatrics seek to weave this content into medical education and ignite interest in the field. The Association of Directors of Medical Student Education in Psychiatry's Geriatric Psychiatry Task Force created an online bibliography of peer-reviewed, web-based learning activities in geriatric psychiatry, along with recommendations for where in the 4-year curriculum such content might be delivered.[17] Given the interdisciplinary nature of geriatrics, the development of geriatrics curricula aimed at interprofessional learners is increasingly emphasized and recommended.[18] As one example, Wu and colleagues described teaching "the 4 Ms of older adult health care" using older adult volunteers from the community to participate in Zoom interviews with first-year nursing, medical, and physician associate students.[19]

Geriatrics Interest Groups (GIGs) are an extracurricular method for offering health professional students' educational opportunities, faculty mentorship, and networking with fellow trainees and faculty who share an interest in caring for older adults. Such groups are often sponsored by or affiliated with to national organizations such as the

American Geriatrics Society, which offers free or discounted student memberships including journal subscriptions, annual meeting discounts, Beers Criteria pocket cards, mentorship, and a US$200 annual stipend for programming.[20] Involvement in GIGs promotes interest in geriatrics via faculty mentorship, networking, dispelling stigma, and career advancement.[21] GIGs can also offer opportunities for greater exposure to older adults themselves. For example, van Dyck and colleagues developed and implemented a telephone outreach program aimed at alleviating social isolation of nursing home elders during the pandemic by matching them with GIG student members for weekly friendly phone calls.[22]

Exposure to older adults and to geriatric psychiatrists need not require the creation of formal curricular or extracurricular interventions. Additional considerations should include less formal, yet impactful experiences such as medical student shadowing in the preclinical years or having geriatric psychiatry faculty teach in the preclinical geriatrics or psychiatry curriculum. In schools fortunate enough to have geriatric psychiatrists on faculty, clerkships should optimize the number of students rotating on geriatric psychiatry services and clinics. Geriatric psychiatry faculty can invite medical students to participate in scholarly projects, articles, and community service of older adults. As one example, geriatric psychiatrists included a medical student in the implementation of a weekly online forum for older adult education, peer support, and social engagement during the coronavirus disease (COVID-19) pandemic.[23] Interested medical students should also be encouraged to attend the annual meeting of the AAGP; they are eligible for travel funding through the organization's Scholars Program.[24]

Although virtually all graduating medical students must be prepared to care for older adults with mental health concerns, a significant minority of graduates will enter psychiatry residency and an even smaller minority will pursue geriatric psychiatry as a career. Indeed, medical student interest in psychiatry is on the increase for the 11th consecutive year.[25] Now is an opportune time to introduce geriatric psychiatry to early learners, as both critically important educational content but also a viable, exciting career option.

Residency Education

The growing need for geriatric mental health-care providers combined with the decreasing numbers of trainees completing geriatric psychiatry subspecialty fellowships indicates that most geriatric patients are likely served by general psychiatrists.[3,26,27] Thus, experts agree that psychiatry residency is an important time for trainees to develop both an interest and competence in the mental health care of older adults.[28,29]

The Accreditation Council for Graduate Medical Education (ACGME), the body responsible for accrediting all graduate medical training programs for physicians in the United States, requires 1-month full time equivalent (FTE) of geriatric psychiatry during psychiatry residency.[30] ACGME guidelines detail certain experiences that must be included in this rotation: "diagnosis and management of mental disorders in geriatric patients with coexistent medical disorders; diagnosis and management, including management of the cognitive component, of degenerative disorders; basic neuropsychological testing of cognitive functioning in the elderly; and management of drug interactions."[30] The 1-month FTE requirement for geriatric psychiatry is equivalent to the 1-month FTE requirement for managing substance use disorders but less than the 2-months FTE required for consult-liaison or child and adolescent psychiatry. In addition, although the ACGME requires child and adolescent psychiatry rotations to be supervised by board-certified child and adolescent psychiatrists, no such requirement exists for geriatric psychiatry.

The 1-month FTE geriatric psychiatry requirement is met in many ways across different psychiatry residency programs. In a 2006 survey, psychiatry program directors reported that most residencies use more than one clinical setting to teach geriatric psychiatry, most often inpatient or outpatient.[28] Fewer rotations include exposure to diverse settings highlighting the breadth of geriatric psychiatry: geriatric consultation-liaison, memory clinics, nursing homes, assisted living, home care, hospice care, senior centers, and electroconvulsive therapy.[27,28] The timing of geriatric psychiatry rotations in the United States is also highly variable. A survey of psychiatry residency program directors conducted in 2018 revealed that a plurality (42.7%) of residencies conducted required geriatric psychiatry rotations during the second postgraduate year (PGY). Yet 14.6% of programs conducted required rotations in PGY-1, 24.4% in PGY-3, and another 14.6% in PGY-4.[27] Overall, psychiatry residency program directors in the United States stated the most common duration of a rotation is 4 weeks, consistent with the ACGME minimum.[27] Although psychiatry program directors rated geriatric psychiatry as the third most important curricular topic (after emergency and addiction psychiatry), "competing curricular demands" was identified as the most significant barrier to expanding training in geriatrics.[28]

Most psychiatry residencies offer additional electives in geriatric psychiatry during PGY-4. However, the percentage of residencies offering these electives may be declining. Surveys indicated that 82% of residencies offered electives in geriatrics in 2006, whereas in 2018 only 72.7% of residencies offered electives in geriatrics.[27,28] Given the importance of training in geriatric psychiatry during residency, several groups proposed additional structured opportunities. One group proposed a 6-month geriatric psychiatry "track" during PGY-4, serving as a "mini-fellowship" to include both clinical and didactic experiences for residents who want geriatrics training but do not wish to pursue a fellowship.[26] Although this opportunity could be a good compromise, a survey conducted by this group indicated that 28% of residents with a high interest in fellowship would be less likely to complete fellowship if a track were available.[26] Another alternative proposed by Kirwin and colleagues is to offer residents the opportunity to enter geriatric psychiatry (or consult/liaison or addictions) fellowships during PGY-4 instead of PGY-5 (also known as "fast tracking").[31] The main advantage of reducing the total years of residency and subspecialty training is to reduce time and financial burdens on trainees, which were identified as the major limitations trainees cite in pursuing fellowships.[7,31,32] However, a review of psychiatry residency websites indicated that 99% of residencies have some required rotation in PGY-4, including longitudinal outpatient clinics or administrative and leadership experiences, that would need to be adjusted for residents to pursue fellowships.[33] In 2016, the American Board of Psychiatry and Neurology (ABPN) solicited feedback from multiple stakeholders on the proposal to offer fellowships during PGY-4 but a consensus was not reached and, so far, the proposal has not been adopted.[7]

Few studies have investigated whether residents attain competence in treating older mental health patients, although competence remains low based on the available evidence. A survey of psychiatry residents indicated that only 13% of residents do not wish to pursue subspecialty training because they already feel confident they can treat older patients.[26] A recent survey of Veterans Affairs mental health providers found only modest self-efficacy in treating people living with dementia.[34] Another survey of psychiatry residents at the University of Southern California found that only 13% of PGY-4 residents felt "very well prepared" to address grief in older patients and only 6% felt "very well prepared" to address loneliness.[35]

A recent scoping review summarized novel interventions outside required and elective residency rotations to increase interest and competence in geriatric psychiatry among residents.[36] To improve competence among residents, interventions included a simulation exercise to increase learners' awareness of the physical and cognitive changes in older adults,[37] a 4-page written inpatient geriatric psychiatry primer for residents,[38] and a national educational study-group program in Canada.[39] More recently, the AAGP COVID-19 Online Trainee Curriculum (aagponline.org/covidcurriculum) was developed with a focus on supplementing resident education in geriatric psychiatry during the pandemic. The curriculum contains 33 video lectures by AAGP-member experts on a wide range of geriatric psychiatry topics.[40] The scoping review also identified several factors that led to increased interest in geriatric psychiatry among residents: positive clinical experiences with older adults, positive experiences caring for older adults before medical school, personal relationships with older adults, appreciating the complexity of geriatrics, and the perception of positive qualities among geriatric psychiatry supervisors.[36] The main intervention identified by the scoping review to increase interest among residents to pursue geriatric psychiatry was the AAGP Scholars Program, which was developed in 2010 and funded by the AAGP membership.[24] Nearly two-thirds of Scholars Program participants decide to pursue geriatric psychiatry fellowship, and 88.9% of participants report the program influenced career decision-making.[24,41,42] Among Scholars Program participants, attending more than one AAGP annual meeting, maintaining AAGP membership, and meeting potential collaborators through the Scholars Program were the most important factors affecting the decision to pursue fellowship,[42] suggesting that one strategy to improve recruitment to the field is to facilitate trainees' involvement in the AAGP.

For the future, the literature supports many approaches may be used by geriatric psychiatrists and general psychiatrists at their home institutions to increase interest in geriatric psychiatry during residency. Examples include collaborating with residents on scholarly projects related to geriatric psychiatry,[42] referring residents to the AAGP Scholars Program (or donating to support Scholars),[42] promoting earlier exposure to geriatric psychiatry during residency,[43] and facilitating positive experiences with older adult mental health patients.[43]

FELLOWSHIP EDUCATION

Geriatric psychiatry fellowship is a 1-year advanced graduate medical education clinical training opportunity offered after the completion of a general psychiatry residency. According to the ACGME, "geriatric psychiatry focuses on the prevention, diagnosis, evaluation, and treatment of psychiatric disorders seen in older adult patients."[44] An educational program in geriatric psychiatry must be organized to provide "professional knowledge, skills, and opportunities to develop competence through a well-supervised clinical experience."[44] The ACGME competencies delineate program requirements specific to geriatric psychiatry: each program must integrate training related to the comprehensive care and treatment of older adults, which includes the diagnosis and treatment of psychiatric, cognitive and associated neuropsychiatric illness, the mental status examination, incorporating cognitive screening, functional, medical and caregiver assessment, as well as the identification of elder abuse.[44] Guidelines further elucidate the medical knowledge required for fellows, from the complex interface of the biological and social factors that affect older adults to changes in pharmacokinetics and pharmacodynamics that impact drug metabolism.[44]

There are also clear requirements related to the type of clinical experiences fellows must engage in during their training, including longitudinal patient care and geriatric psychiatry consultation, participation on an interdisciplinary treatment team and a minimum of 2 hours of faculty preceptorship weekly.[44] In practice, programs typically offer a range of opportunities in nursing home care, inpatient geriatric psychiatry, outpatient longitudinal geriatric psychiatry, consultation-liaison in the acute hospital setting as well as in a variety of other settings such as consultative work in hospice, palliative care and primary care settings, electroconvulsive therapy, neurology clinics (eg, movement disorders, neurocognitive/memory care, and stroke clinics), sleep clinic, research settings, elder abuse agencies, community care settings, geriatric medicine clinics, and home visits (**Table 1**). Exposure to these myriad opportunities provides fellows with a broad educational experience allowing them to better inform their postgraduation career path and prepare them for the complexities of providing care to older adult patients across a spectrum of settings.

Learning to provide care to patients on an interdisciplinary team is essential to the care of older adult patients and, as noted above, an ACGME requirement.[44] Many programs require the provision of care alongside social work, case management, nurses (both registered nurses and advanced practice nurses), pharmacy, neuropsychology, and occupational and physical therapy. These teams expand beyond the confines of the clinic setting and may include a patient's family

Table 1
Hospital settings and multidisciplinary collaborators in geriatric psychiatry fellowship training

Care Setting	Rotation Opportunities	Team Collaborators
Inpatient	Inpatient geriatric psychiatry Consult-liaison Interventional psychiatry (ECT) Palliative care/hospice	Social work Nurses (RN and APRN) Pharmacists Occupational and physical therapists Inpatient medical services (internal medicine, neurology) Neuropsychology Family/conservator
Outpatient	Outpatient longitudinal geriatric psychiatry Neurology clinics (movement disorders, neurocognitive/memory care, stroke clinics) Sleep clinic Geriatric medicine clinics Home visits Interventional psychiatry (ECT, rTMS, ketamine) Clinical research settings Elder abuse agencies	Social work Case management Nurses (RN and APRN) Neuropsychology Visiting nurse agencies Home health-care attendants Adult day care Research assistants Family/conservator
Long-term care settings (ie, nursing home, assisted living facility, rest home)	Onsite nursing home consultation Outpatient assessment of LTC patients in longitudinal geriatric psychiatry clinics	Nurses (RN and APRN) Occupational and physical therapists Long-term care staff Onsite medical team members (MD, PA, APRN) Family/conservator

Abbreviations: APRN, advanced practice registered nurse; ECT, electroconvulsive therapy; LTC, long term care; MD, medical doctor; PA, physician's assistant; rTMS, repetitive transcranial magnetic stimulation; RN, registered nurse.

members and/or close friends, visiting nurse agencies, home health-care attendants, and adult day care and long-term care staff. Developing the skill set to successfully collaborate in team settings, including clear communication, attention to detail, and leadership are an integral part of the experience during geriatric psychiatry fellowship training.

Programs are also required to provide didactic education and other academic experiences beyond direct patient care.[44] Didactics may be attended by other learners assigned to geriatric psychiatry during a given time frame, including medical students, general psychiatry and neurology residents, neuropsychology interns, geriatric medicine and palliative care fellows, physician assistant and nurse practitioner trainees, as well as pharmacy residents. The ACGME requires attendance and evaluation of didactic experiences; fellows are obligated to attend 70% of these sessions.[44] Some institutions offer didactic education specifically in neuroimaging, whereas others may offer case-based conferences, journal clubs, fellow-led seminars, as well as morbidity and mortality conferences.

Additionally, geriatric psychiatry fellows typically participate in extracurricular experiences to augment their learning, such as completion of a scholarly project. These projects may include publication of an article, presenting at a national conference, completion of a poster, curricula development, or engagement in a quality improvement initiative. Moreover, some institutions with available financial support may provide funding for fellows to attend the AAGP annual meeting. This provides trainees exposure to our field on a national level, allows them to access mentorship outside of their home institution, offers the opportunity to meet with prospective employers and consider mechanisms for future engagement in the organization through participation in subcommittees and junior leadership positions.

Very importantly, geriatric psychiatry training offers multiple opportunities to serve as a mentor, educator, and role model for junior trainees (medical, physician assistant, nursing, and pharmacy students and residents) as well as for peer colleagues, including geriatric medicine and palliative care fellows. These interactions, in the case of junior trainees, can inspire interest in the care of older adult patients. Fellows may encourage junior trainees to participate in research projects, attend an AAGP annual meeting through the Scholars program, or foster interest in a potential career in geriatric psychiatry through informal discussion and shared engagement in patient care.

Aside from many of the formal requirements and informal initiatives outlined previously, one of the tasks of fellowship programs is to strongly encourage fellows to take the board examination on completion of training. The requirements for ABPN board certification in geriatric psychiatry include the completion of ACGME accredited training, a valid and unrestricted medical license, and passing a 200 item multiple choice examination spanning topics across many domains, including aging (developmental, biological, psychological, and social), psychopathology and psychiatric diagnosis, diagnostic methods, the interface of medicine and psychiatry, and the neurologic and neuropsychiatric aspects of aging.[7] The examination is offered every 2 years. As of December 2021, 3638 candidates received certificates for completion of the ABPN subspecialty examination.[45] Between the years 2017 to 2021, 172 board eligible geriatric psychiatrists took the examination and 165 passed, notably a 96% pass rate.[46] Unfortunately, although, these numbers indicate that many who complete fellowship, do not in fact sit for the board examination.

Beginning in 2022, the maintenance of certification requirements for geriatric psychiatry was modified.[47] Previously, board certified geriatric psychiatrists were required to pass 2 examinations every 10 years: one in general psychiatry and a second in geriatric psychiatry. With the new iteration, those wishing to maintain dual certification must complete 50 topic articles (30 in general psychiatry, 20 in geriatric psychiatry) every 3 years.[47] The hope is that this approach allows for more evidence-based acquisition of knowledge on a longitudinal basis, as well as encourages more geriatric psychiatrists to maintain their board certification status.

GERIATRIC PSYCHIATRY FOR GENERAL PSYCHIATRISTS

For those in general psychiatry practice seeking additional educational opportunities in geriatric psychiatry, the AAGP offers an online COVID-19 curriculum with free access to all (www.aagponline.org/covidcurriculum), which provides 33 online content-based modules on a variety of salient topics including geriatric assessment, normal aging, delirium, late-life depression, and the most common dementias.[40] To date, 519 unique users accessed the curriculum. The AAGP meeting, offered annually in March, is another opportunity for general psychiatrists to deepen their knowledge base. Aside from the annual meeting, the AAGP offers live webinars approximately monthly; these webinars are recorded for future viewing as well. Finally, systems-based programs such as VA's Ask the Expert-Geriatric Psychiatry program are available to those requiring patient consultation in the VA system.[48] Given the growing older demographic of our population and the declining number of geriatric psychiatrists, this type of system-specific consultation model will likely become more common in the future.

DIVERSITY, EQUITY, AND INCLUSION IN GERIATRIC PSYCHIATRY TRAINING

Given the increasing diversity of the older adult population as well as the increasing diversity of medical trainees, it behooves all involved in geriatric psychiatry training to strive for equitable and inclusive clinical care and learning environments. Both LCME and ACGME standards require the inclusion of curricula on culturally competent care for undergraduate and graduate medical education, respectively.[8,30] The past decade has witnessed significant growth in published literature at the interface of medical education and diversity, equity, and inclusion, related to both patients and trainees. With regard to patient care, Joo and colleagues described the various training needs of geriatric mental health providers to prepare them to competently care for a diverse older adult population.[49] With regard to trainee education, MedEd-PORTAL, the AAMC's journal of teaching and learning resources in the health professions, has a collection of curricula dedicated to "Anti-Racism in Medicine" with more than 35 published learning modules, with topics ranging from structural competency to responding to microaggressions.[50]

One such antiracism learning module, entitled ERASE, has been applied to training in geriatric psychiatry.[51] This interactive workshop is designed to help participants manage mistreatment by patients (eg, racism, microaggressions, problematic "compliments").[52] The ERASE framework includes: *E*xpect and prepare for mistreatment, *R*ecognize mistreatment, *A*ddress mistreatment in real time, *S*eek support/*S*upport the targeted individual, and *E*stablish a positive culture. Given generational differences and potential for cognitive impairment, geriatric psychiatrists and trainees are likely to encounter mistreatment by patients, either as recipients or bystanders. Preparing faculty and trainees to intervene and support each other in these instances is crucial for promoting inclusive learning and clinical care environments.

SUMMARY

Geriatric psychiatry training is dynamic, interactive, diverse, team-oriented, and allows psychiatrists to practice at the interface of psychiatry, medicine, and neurology.

Yet the number of geriatric psychiatrists is decreasing at the same time the population of older adults suffering from cognitive and mental illnesses is increasing. Thus, the psychiatric needs of older adults will increasingly be addressed by general psychiatrists and other physicians. Official standards for medical schools do not require specific education in geriatric psychiatry, and although psychiatry residencies are required to provide 1 month of geriatric psychiatry education, competency is rarely achieved. Nonetheless, implementing evidence-formed curricula exist to improve knowledge and skills and to inspire more trainees to consider a career in the mental health care of older adults is tenable across all levels of medical education.

CLINICS CARE POINTS

- Current medical student and resident education is insufficient to address the complex care of older adult psychiatric patients.
- Enhanced learning opportunities in medical school and psychiatry residency serve 2 vital purposes: improve the knowledge base for future general psychiatrists and provide exposure to geriatric psychiatry with the goal of recruitment into the field.
- Evidence-informed curricular and extracurricular geriatric psychiatry interventions exist, although their implementation is contingent on resources, including geriatric psychiatry faculty and curricular time.

DISCLOSURE

Drs M.L. Conroy, K.M. Wilkins, L.I. van Dyck, and B.C. Yarns do not have any disclosures to report.

REFERENCES

1. Vincent GK, Velkoff VA. The next four decades: the older population in the United States: 2010 to 2050. US Department of Commerce, Economics and Statistics Administration, US Census Bureau. 2010. Available at: https://www.census.gov/prod/2010pubs/p25-1138.pdf. Accessed April 1, 2022.
2. Ortman JM, Velkoff VA, Hogan H. An aging nation: the older population in the United States. Washington, DC: United States Census Bureau; 2014.
3. Committee on the Mental Health Workforce for Geriatric Populations, Board on Health Care Services, Institute of Medicine. Assessing the service needs of older adults with mental health and substance use conditions. In: Eden J, Maslow K, Le M, et al, editors. The mental health and substance use workforce for older adults: in whose hands? Washington, DC: National Academies Press; 2012. p. 39–139.
4. Chiriboga DA, Hernandez M. Multicultural competence in geropsychology. In: APA handbook of clinical geropsychology, Vol. 1: history and status of the field and perspectives on aging. Washington, DC: American Psychological Association; 2015. p. 379–419.
5. National Resident Matching Program (NRMP). Main Residency Match Data and Reports. 2022. Available at: https://www.nrmp.org/match-data-analytics/residency-data-reports/. Accessed May 10, 2022.
6. Accreditation Council for Graduate Medical Education (ACGME). Number of accredited programs and on-duty residents for the academic year by specialty.

2022. Available at: https://apps.acgme-i.org/ads/Public/Reports/Report/3. Accessed May 4, 2022.

7. Juul D, Colenda CC, Lyness JM, et al. Subspecialty Training and Certification in Geriatric Psychiatry: A 25-Year Overview. Am J Geriatr Psychiatry 2017;25(5): 445–53.

8. Liaison Committee on Medical Education (LCME). Functions and structure of a medical school: Standards for accreditation for medical education programs leading to the MD degree. 2022. Available at: https://lcme.org/publications/. Accessed April 11, 2022.

9. Leipzig RM, Granville L, Simpson D, et al. Keeping granny safe on July 1: a consensus on minimum geriatrics competencies for graduating medical students. Acad Med 2009;84(5):604–10.

10. Tinetti M, Huang A, Molnar F. The Geriatrics 5M's: A New Way of Communicating What We Do. J Am Geriatr Soc 2017;65(9):2115.

11. Association of Directors of Geriatrics Academic Programs (ADGAP). Geriatrics competencies for medical students. Available at: https://adgap. americangeriatrics.org/education-training/competencies/geriatrics-competencies-medical-students2021. Accessed April 8, 2022.

12. Lehmann SW, Brooks WB, Popeo D, et al. Development of geriatric mental health learning objectives for medical students: a response to the institute of medicine 2012 report. Am J Geriatr Psychiatry 2017;25(10):1041–7.

13. Wilkins KM, Blazek MC, Brooks WB, et al. Six things all medical students need to know about geriatric psychiatry (and how to teach them). Acad Psychiatry 2017; 41(5):693–700.

14. Lehmann SW, Blazek MC, Popeo DM. Geriatric psychiatry in the psychiatry clerkship: a survey of current education practices. Acad Psychiatry 2015;39(3):312–5.

15. American Board of Psychiatry and Neurology (ABPN). 2019 annual report. 2019. Available at: https://www.abpn.com/wp-content/uploads/2020/05/ABPN_2019_Annual_Report.pdf. Accessed April 11, 2022.

16. Wilkins KM, Wagenaar D, Brooks WB. Emerging trends in undergraduate medical education: implications for geriatric psychiatry. Am J Geriatr Psychiatry 2018; 26(5):610–3.

17. Blazek MC, Wagenaar DB, Brooks WB, et al. Filling the gap in geriatric psychiatry education for medical students: development of the ADMSEP annotated bibliography of web-based resources on geriatric mental health for medical student education. Acad Psychiatry 2021;45(4):517–20.

18. Farrell TW, Luptak MK, Supiano KP, et al. State of the science: interprofessional approaches to aging, dementia, and mental health. J Am Geriatr Soc 2018; 66(Suppl 1):S40–7.

19. Wu BJ, Honan L, Tinetti ME, et al. The virtual 4Ms: A novel curriculum for first year health professional students during COVID-19. J Am Geriatr Soc 2021;69(6): E13–6.

20. American Geriatrics Society (AGS). Student Membership. 2022. Available at: https://www.americangeriatrics.org/membership/benefits/student-membership. Accessed April 8, 2022.

21. Perrella A, Cuperfain AB, Canfield AB, et al. Do Interest Groups Cultivate Interest? Trajectories of Geriatric Interest Group Members. Can Geriatr J 2020; 23(3):264–9.

22. van Dyck LI, Wilkins KM, Ouellet J, et al. Combating Heightened Social Isolation of Nursing Home Elders: The Telephone Outreach in the COVID-19 Outbreak Program. Am J Geriatr Psychiatry 2020;28(9):989–92.

23. van Dyck L, Wilkins K, Mecca M, et al. Social connections for seniors during COVID-19: An online psychoeducation and peer support program. Am J Geriatr Psychiatry 2021;29(4):S135.

24. Wilkins KM, Forester B, Conroy M, et al. The American Association for Geriatric Psychiatry's Scholars Program: A Model Program for Recruitment into Psychiatric Subspecialties. Acad Psychiatry 2017;41(5):688–92.

25. Moran M. Psychiatry match numbers increase for 11th straight year. Psychiatric News. 2022. Available at: https://psychnews.psychiatryonline.org/doi/10.1176/appi.pn.2022.05.5.24. Accessed April 25, 2022.

26. Duffy S, Schultz SK, Maixner S, et al. Meeting Residents Halfway: the Geriatric Psychiatry Residency Track. Acad Psychiatry 2019;43(1):142–3.

27. Conroy ML, Meyen RA, Slade MD, et al. Predictors for Matriculation into Geriatric Psychiatry Fellowship: Data from a 2019-2020 National Survey of U.S. Program Directors. Acad Psychiatry 2021;45(4):435–9.

28. Warshaw GA, Bragg EJ, Layde JB, et al. Geriatrics education in psychiatric residencies: a national survey of program directors. Acad Psychiatry 2010;34(1):39–45.

29. Camp MM, Palka JM, Duong K, et al. Psychiatry resident education in neurocognitive disorders: a national survey of program directors in psychiatry. Acad Psychiatry 2022;46(1):120–7.

30. Accreditation Council for Graduate Medical Education (ACGME). ACGME Program Requirements for Graduate Medical Education in Psychiatry. 2021. Available at: https://www.acgme.org/globalassets/pfassets/programrequirements/400_psychiatry_2021.pdf. Accessed April 6, 2022.

31. Kirwin P, Conroy M, Lyketsos C, et al. A call to restructure psychiatry general and subspecialty training. Acad Psychiatry 2016;40(1):145–8.

32. Lieff SJ, Tolomiczenko GS, Dunn LB. Effect of training and other influences on the development of career interest in geriatric psychiatry. Am J Geriatr Psychiatry 2003;11(3):300–8.

33. Vestal HS, Belitsky R, Bernstein CA, et al. Required and Elective Experiences During the 4th Year: An Analysis of ACGME Accredited Psychiatry Residency Program Websites. Acad Psychiatry 2016;40(5):816–20.

34. Wyman MF, Voils CI, Trivedi R, et al. Perspectives of Veterans Affairs mental health providers on working with older adults with dementia and their caregivers. Gerontol Geriatr Educ 2021;42(1):114–25.

35. Winthrop M, Feil D. Psychiatric resident perceptions of competency in the management of social isolation and grief in geriatric patients. Am J Geriatr Psychiatry 2022;30(4):S96–7.

36. Hernandez CR, Camp MME. Current educational practices for major neurocognitive disorders in psychiatry: a scoping review. Acad Psychiatry 2021;45(4):451–9.

37. de Abreu ID, Hinojosa-Lindsey M, Asghar-Ali AA. A simulation exercise to raise learners' awareness of the physical and cognitive changes in older adults. Acad Psychiatry 2017;41(5):684–7.

38. Thomas NA, Van Enkevort E, Garrett RK. Camp MME. geriatric psychiatry inpatient primer for residents. Acad Psychiatry 2019;43(6):585–9.

39. Law M, Rapoport MJ, Seitz D, et al. Evaluation of a National Online Educational Program in Geriatric Psychiatry. Acad Psychiatry 2016;40(6):923–7.

40. Conroy ML, Garcia-Pittman EC, Ali H, et al. The COVID-19 AAGP Online Trainee Curriculum: Development and Method of Initial Evaluation. Am J Geriatr Psychiatry 2020;28(9):1004–8.

41. Wilkins KM, Conroy ML, Yarns BC, et al. The American Association for Geriatric Psychiatry's Trainee Programs: Participant Characteristics and Perceived Benefits. Am J Geriatr Psychiatry 2020;28(11):1156–63.
42. Conroy ML, Yarns BC, Wilkins KM, et al. The AAGP scholars program: predictors of pursuing geriatric psychiatry fellowship training. Am J Geriatr Psychiatry 2020; 29(4):365–74.
43. Rej S, Laliberté V, Rapoport MJ, et al. What makes residents interested in geriatric psychiatry? A pan-Canadian online survey of psychiatry residents. Am J Geriatr Psychiatry 2015;23(7):735–43.
44. Accreditation Council for Graduate Medical Education (ACGME). ACGME program requirements for graduate medical education in geriatric psychiatry. 2022. Available at: https://www.acgme.org/globalassets/pfassets/programrequirements/407_geriatricpsychiatry_2022_tcc.pdf. Accessed April 28, 2022.
45. American Board of Psychiatry and Neurology (ABPN). Facts and Statistics. 2022. Available at: https://www.abpn.com/about/facts-and-statistics/. Accessed April 28, 2022.
46. American Board of Psychiatry and Neurology (ABPN). Pass Rates for First-time Takers. 2021. Available at: https://www.abpn.com/wp-content/uploads/2022/02/ABPN-Pass-Rates-First-time-Taker-5-year-2021.pdf. Accessed April 28, 2022.
47. American Boardof Psychiatry and Neurology (ABPN). New Article-Based Continuing Certification (ABCC) Pathway. 2022. Available at: https://www.abpn.com/maintain-certification/article-based-continuing-certification-abcc-pathway/. Accessed May 10, 2022.
48. Padala P, Schultz S, Khatkhate G, et al. Ask The Expert Geriatric Psychiatry: VA program to support clinicians. Am J Geriatr Psychiatry 2022;30(4):S18.
49. Joo JH, Jimenez DE, Xu J, et al. Perspectives on training needs for geriatric mental health providers: preparing to serve a diverse older adult population. Am J Geriatr Psychiatry 2019;27(7):728–36.
50. MedEdPORTAL. Anti-racism in medicine collection. 2022. Available at: https://www.mededportal.org/anti-racism. Accessed May 6, 2022.
51. Wilkins KM, Goldenberg MN, Cyrus KD, et al. Addressing mistreatment by patients in geriatric subspecialties: a new framework. Am J Geriatr Psychiatry 2022;30(1):78–86.
52. Wilkins KM, Goldenberg MN, Cyrus KD. ERASE-ing patient mistreatment of trainees: faculty workshop. MedEdPORTAL 2019;15:10865.

UNITED STATES POSTAL SERVICE®

Statement of Ownership, Management, and Circulation
(All Periodicals Publications Except Requester Publications)

1. Publication Title	2. Publication Number	3. Filing Date
PSYCHIATRIC CLINICS OF NORTH AMERICA	000 – 703	9/18/2022

4. Issue Frequency	5. Number of Issues Published Annually	6. Annual Subscription Price
MAR, JUN, SEP, DEC	4	$345.00

7. Complete Mailing Address of Known Office of Publication (Not printer) (Street, city, county, state, and ZIP+4®)

ELSEVIER INC.
230 Park Avenue, Suite 800
New York, NY 10169

Contact Person
Malathi Samayan

Telephone (Include area code)
91-44-4299-4507

8. Complete Mailing Address of Headquarters or General Business Office of Publisher (Not printer)

ELSEVIER INC.
230 Park Avenue, Suite 800
New York, NY 10169

9. Full Names and Complete Mailing Addresses of Publisher, Editor, and Managing Editor (Do not leave blank)

Publisher (Name and complete mailing address)

DOLORES MELONI, ELSEVIER INC.
1600 JOHN F KENNEDY BLVD. SUITE 1800
MEGAN ASHDOWN, PA 19103-2899

Editor (Name and complete mailing address)

MEGAN ASHDOWN, ELSEVIER INC.
1600 JOHN F KENNEDY BLVD. SUITE 1800
PHILADELPHIA, PA 19103-2899

Managing Editor (Name and complete mailing address)

PATRICK MANLEY, ELSEVIER INC.
1600 JOHN F KENNEDY BLVD. SUITE 1800
PHILADELPHIA, PA 19103-2899

10. Owner (Do not leave blank. If the publication is owned by a corporation, give the name and address of the corporation immediately followed by the names and addresses of all stockholders owning or holding 1 percent or more of the total amount of stock. If not owned by a corporation, give the names and addresses of the individual owners. If owned by a partnership or other unincorporated firm, give its name and address as well as those of each individual owner. If the publication is published by a nonprofit organization, give its name and address.)

Full Name	Complete Mailing Address
WHOLLY OWNED SUBSIDIARY OF REED/ELSEVIER, US HOLDINGS	1600 JOHN F KENNEDY BLVD. SUITE 1800 PHILADELPHIA, PA 19103-2899

11. Known Bondholders, Mortgagees, and Other Security Holders Owning or Holding 1 Percent or More of Total Amount of Bonds, Mortgages, or Other Securities. If none, check box ▶ ☐ None

Full Name	Complete Mailing Address
N/A	

12. Tax Status (For completion by nonprofit organizations authorized to mail at nonprofit rates) (Check one)
The purpose, function, and nonprofit status of this organization and the exempt status for federal income tax purposes:
☒ Has Not Changed During Preceding 12 Months
☐ Has Changed During Preceding 12 Months (Publisher must submit explanation of change with this statement)

PS Form 3526, July 2014 (Page 1 of 4 (see instructions page 4)) PSN: 7530-01-000-9931   PRIVACY NOTICE: See our privacy policy on www.usps.com.

13. Publication Title	14. Issue Date for Circulation Data Below
PSYCHIATRIC CLINICS OF NORTH AMERICA	JUNE 2022

15. Extent and Nature of Circulation			Average No. Copies Each Issue During Preceding 12 Months	No. Copies of Single Issue Published Nearest to Filing Date
a. Total Number of Copies (Net press run)			204	160
b. Paid Circulation (By Mail and Outside the Mail)	(1)	Mailed Outside-County Paid Subscriptions Stated on PS Form 3541 (Include paid distribution above nominal rate, advertiser's proof copies, and exchange copies)	98	81
	(2)	Mailed In-County Paid Subscriptions Stated on PS Form 3541 (Include paid distribution above nominal rate, advertiser's proof copies, and exchange copies)	0	0
	(3)	Paid Distribution Outside the Mails Including Sales Through Dealers and Carriers, Street Vendors, Counter Sales, and Other Paid Distribution Outside USPS®	65	50
	(4)	Paid Distribution by Other Classes of Mail Through the USPS (e.g., First-Class Mail®)	0	0
c. Total Paid Distribution (Sum of 15b (1), (2), (3), and (4))		▶	163	131
d. Free or Nominal Rate Distribution (By Mail and Outside the Mail)	(1)	Free or Nominal Rate Outside-County Copies included on PS Form 3541	25	13
	(2)	Free or Nominal Rate In-County Copies included on PS Form 3541	0	0
	(3)	Free or Nominal Rate Copies Mailed at Other Classes Through the USPS (e.g., First-Class Mail)	0	0
	(4)	Free or Nominal Rate Distribution Outside the Mail (Carriers or other means)	0	0
e. Total Free or Nominal Rate Distribution (Sum of 15d (1), (2), (3) and (4))		▶	25	13
f. Total Distribution (Sum of 15c and 15e)		▶	188	144
g. Copies not Distributed (See Instructions to Publishers #4 (page #3))		▶	16	16
h. Total (Sum of 15f and g)		▶	204	160
i. Percent Paid (15c divided by 15f times 100)		▶	86.7%	90.97%

* If you are claiming electronic copies, go to line 16 on page 3. If you are not claiming electronic copies, skip to line 17 on page 3.

16. Electronic Copy Circulation

	Average No. Copies Each Issue During Preceding 12 Months	No. Copies of Single Issue Published Nearest to Filing Date
a. Paid Electronic Copies ▶		
b. Total Paid Print Copies (Line 15c) + Paid Electronic Copies (Line 16a) ▶		
c. Total Print Distribution (Line 15f) + Paid Electronic Copies (Line 16a) ▶		
d. Percent Paid (Both Print & Electronic Copies) (16b divided by 16c × 100) ▶		

☒ I certify that 50% of all my distributed copies (electronic and print) are paid above a nominal price.

17. Publication of Statement of Ownership
☒ If the publication is a general publication, publication of this statement is required. Will be printed in the DECEMBER 2022 issue of this publication.   ☐ Publication not required.

18. Signature and Title of Editor, Publisher, Business Manager, or Owner

Malathi Samayan

Malathi Samayan - Distribution Controller

Date 9/18/2022

I certify that all information furnished on this form is true and complete. I understand that anyone who furnishes false or misleading information on this form or who omits material or information requested on the form may be subject to criminal sanctions (including fines and imprisonment) and/or civil sanctions (including civil penalties).

PS Form 3526, July 2014 (Page 3 of 4)   PRIVACY NOTICE: See our privacy policy on www.usps.com.

Moving?

Make sure your subscription moves with you!

To notify us of your new address, find your **Clinics Account Number** (located on your mailing label above your name), and contact customer service at:

Email: journalscustomerservice-usa@elsevier.com

800-654-2452 (subscribers in the U.S. & Canada)
314-447-8871 (subscribers outside of the U.S. & Canada)

Fax number: 314-447-8029

Elsevier Health Sciences Division
Subscription Customer Service
3251 Riverport Lane
Maryland Heights, MO 63043

*To ensure uninterrupted delivery of your subscription, please notify us at least 4 weeks in advance of move.

Printed and bound by CPI Group (UK) Ltd, Croydon, CR0 4YY

03/10/2024

01040467-0016